Developmental Co-ordination Disorder in Adults

SHARON DREW DipCOT

Independent Consultant Occupational Therapist

JENNIFER CREEK

Consultant Editor in Occupational Therapy

W
WHURR PUBLISHERS
LONDON AND PHILADELPHIA

© 2005 Whurr Publishers Ltd (a subsidiary of John Wiley & Sons, Ltd)
First published 2005 by
Whurr Publishers Ltd
The Atrium, Southern Gate, Chichester, West Sussex, PO19 8SQ, U.K
Telephone: (+44) 1243 779777
E-mail: cs-books@wiley.co.uk
Visit our Home page on www.wiley.com

British Library Cataloguing in Publication Data

A catalogue record for this book
is available from the British Library.

ISBN 1 86156 462 7

Coventry University

Typeset by Adrian McLaughlin, a@microguides.net
Printed and bound in the UK by TJ International Ltd, Padstow,
Cornwall, UK.

Contents

Acknowledgements

There are always many people to whom a vote of thanks is needed in a project such as this, but special thanks go to the team at the Dyscovery Centre, which includes staff both past and present, for all the knowledge shared over the years. To Mary Colley and her tireless work in promoting and supporting adults with DCD and related conditions.

My deepest thanks go to Martin my partner, my dad, brother and sister-in-law who have been there for me through a very sad and difficult year.

For my mum xx.

Preface

In 1997, a Centre was opened in Cardiff, South Wales, to provide a comprehensive service for children and young people with specific learning difficulties, and predominantly developmental co-ordination disorder (DCD), sometimes referred to as dyspraxia.

As the team began its work, they realized that DCD was not restricted to childhood but that it was a changing condition that continues to affect individuals into adulthood. It became evident that the needs of the adult with DCD were different from those of the child. Although difficulties with co-ordination and motor skills still existed to some degree, the major areas of difficulty for many adults were organizational skills, time management and short-term memory. These difficulties affected their everyday lives and impacted upon their ability to successfully complete further/higher education, obtain and maintain employment, as well as managing their home.

This book has been written by an occupational therapist who has extensive experience of working with adults and young people with DCD and related conditions. It is a textbook that provides readers with an insight into DCD in adulthood and the impact it has on everyday life. Potential areas of difficulty are outlined, together with potential solutions and strategies that can be utilized by individuals to improve their personal, social and working lives.

Introduction

The study of developmental co-ordination disorder (DCD), also known as dyspraxia, is in relative terms still in its infancy compared to other conditions such as dyslexia and attention deficit/hyperactivity disorder. Nevertheless, a substantial amount of descriptive and experimental work is beginning to emerge. However, much of this work is published in psychological and medical journals, with little in journals devoted to a wider readership.

For many individuals with mild developmental co-ordination disorder (DCD/dyspraxia) the outcome in adulthood is good as many of them learn to compensate for their difficulties, but those with moderate to severe difficulties in childhood continue to struggle with living and learning tasks as adults. Many professionals working within the health and social services believe that DCD is something that children 'grow out of' in time. The reality is, however, that many individuals with DCD continue to have difficulty with a lot of things that most of the general population take for granted in their everyday lives, such as organization of themselves and their belongings, time management and food preparation. These issues may appear to be fairly insignificant to those who are competent, but the impact for individuals with DCD is that these can act as barriers to becoming successful adults in all areas of life: home, personal relationships, work, social life, college and/or university. Research also suggests that the impact of these difficulties over time results in increased risk of mental health problems.

Developmental co-ordination disorder in adults is widespread. Up to 10 per cent of the population are affected by it to some extent, 2–4 per cent severely. However, there is very little awareness and recognition of this condition in adults among the relevant professionals. It is important that the condition is acknowledged and that appropriate support can be accessed by the individual in order to receive a correct diagnosis and thereby receive the help and support they need. This support may also enable the adult with DCD to obtain benefits to which they are entitled, such as Disability Living Allowance, Student Disability Allowance and Access to Work support.

Within this contextual framework and that of current international research, this book sets out to explore the issues which an adult with DCD experiences within the home, in a learning environment such as a college or university, in the workplace and 'at play'.

The book begins by considering the term DCD and its co-existence with other specific learning difficulties. The author examines issues around identification, 'assessment' and intervention, and reflects upon the implications of the diagnosis or 'the label' being given.

In subsequent chapters the author describes how the individual is affected across a range of living and learning activities, such as in the workplace, as an adult learner in college/university, at home and at play. Practical solutions will also be offered for the reader.

The book aims to encourage the reader to consider the individual with DCD as a person who experiences functional difficulties in everyday life where many of the issues can be remediated by practical solutions, rather than having a medical condition which needs to be 'treated'.

CHAPTER 1

What is developmental co-ordination disorder (DCD)?

Issues surrounding nomenclature

Developmental co-ordination disorder (DCD) has only received concentrated attention from researchers in the past 20 years, and as such, longitudinal investigations are only just beginning to be published. Therefore in order to gain a perspective of the manifestations and course of DCD together with its presentation in adulthood, it is necessary to begin by considering the evidence relating to children.

Description (International Consensus Statement – London, Ontario, 1994)

> DCD is a chronic and usually permanent condition characterized by impairment of both functional performance and quality of movement that is not explicable in terms of age or intellect, or by any other diagnosable neurological or psychiatric features.
>
> Individuals with DCD display a qualitative difference in movement which differentiates them from those of the same age without the disability. The nature of these qualitative differences, whilst considered to change over time, tends to persist through the life span. (Fox and Polatajko, 1994, p. 1)

The research that has investigated developmental movement problems has been plagued by a lack of consensus on two fundamental issues (1) the name of the disability and (2) the definition of the disability (Dewey and Wilson, 2001).

The presenting features of motor inco-ordination have been described in the neurological literature for some eighty or more years. Over the years numerous terms have been used to describe individuals with movement skill problems, such as clumsy, awkward and maladroit (Missiuna and Polatajko, 1995). In his comprehensive study, Gubbay (1995) used

1

the term 'clumsiness' for the impairment, which he viewed as a general condition. Gubbay defined it as an impaired ability to perform skilled and purposeful movements by children who are otherwise 'mentally normal' and without 'bodily deformity'.

Historical perspective of nomenclature

1900	Congenital maladroitness (Ford, 1966)
1925	Motor weakness or psychomotor syndrome (Cermak, 1985)
1930	Disorders in praxis due to pyramidal, extra pyramidal or cerebellar dysfunction (Orton, 1937)
1970	Developmental dyspraxia (Ayres, 1972a, 1972b, 1979, 1985)
1975	Clumsy child (Gubbay, 1975)
1980	Beginning to distinguish between different forms of motor dysfunction (David et al., 1981; Cermak, 1985; Sugden and Keogh, 1990)
1992	Specific developmental disorder of motor function introduced (ICD 10) (WHO, 1992)
1994	Developmental co-ordination disorder (DSM IV, APA, 1994)

Although DCD has been proposed as the term used to describe a collection of motor dysfunctions, there remains confusion and inconsistency in the different diagnostic terms used (see table above). Professionals from different backgrounds may use the terms differently. In a study by Missiuna and Polatajko (1995), an examination of available literature found that there were four terms most commonly used, i.e. clumsy child syndrome, sensory integrative dysfunction, developmental dyspraxia and developmental co-ordination disorder.

'Developmental dyspraxia' has been the term most frequently used by various disciplines in the United Kingdom and United States. This term was derived from adult neurology and is more specifically used by neurologists (Denckla, 1984; Denckla and Roeltgen, 1992), occupational therapists (Cermak, 1985; Missiuna and Polatajko, 1995) and neuropsychologists (Dewey, 1995), to describe the motor learning and planning problems experienced by children. These motor planning problems were considered to be due to difficulty integrating information from bodily senses (Ayres, 1980; Cermak, 1991) or to problems with motor sequencing and selection.

Denckla and Roeltgen (1992) defined developmental dyspraxia as a 'disorder of gesture' that includes meaningful or non-meaningful acts. Although this term has been used interchangeably with DCD some feel that 'dyspraxia' is more a specific term related in particular to the organization of movement and/or motor planning. However, clarification of the definition of, and consensus about, the diagnostic criteria for developmental dyspraxia are difficult, given the various usages by a diverse group of professionals and parents (Peters et al., 2001).

The London Consensus Statement referred to earlier offers a clearer and more descriptive definition. It also comments on requirements for assessment and suggestions on identification and intervention techniques. The Consensus further recommended that the term DCD should be used as a key word in publications and literature in order to facilitate interagency review and accessibility.

In a discussion meeting in 1998 at the Novartis Foundation, a number of professionals in the field explored DCD and debated the issues of how to define it, and what it is and what it is not. The general consensus was that the term DCD should be used as an umbrella term with a number of emerging subtypes.

The frequent name changes of the condition reflect an important issue, that the underlying reasons for motor co-ordination difficulties is still not yet fully understood.

Diagnostic criteria

In London, Ontario in 1994, a multi-disciplinary consensus meeting of internationally recognized researchers who worked with children with motor clumsiness, agreed to use the term 'Developmental Co-ordination Disorder' (Fox and Polatajko, 1994) as described in the Diagnostic and Statistical Manual of Mental Disorders, American Psychiatric Association (DSM-IV, 1994).

The DSM-IV Sourcebook, the American Psychiatric Association Diagnostic and Statistical Manual (DSM-IV), outlines the diagnostic features of DCD as being:

Criterion A: A marked impairment in the development of motor co-ordination.

Criterion B: The diagnosis is made only if this impairment significantly interferes with academic achievement or activities of daily living.

Criterion C: The diagnosis is made if the co-ordination difficulties are not due to a general medical condition, e.g. cerebral palsy, muscular dystrophy, and the criteria are not met for Pervasive Developmental Disorder.

Criterion D: If mental retardation is present, the motor difficulties are in excess of those usually associated with it.

Another diagnostic system, the ICD-10 Classification of Mental and Behavioural Disorders in Children and Adolescents (World Health Organization, 1992), uses the term 'Specific Developmental Disorder of Motor Function'.

The main feature of this disorder is a serious impairment of motor co-ordination that is not solely explicable in terms of general intellectual retardation or any specific congenital or acquired neurological disorder (other than the one that may be implicit in the co-ordination abnormality). It is usual for the motor clumsiness to be associated with some degree of impaired performance on visuospatial cognitive tasks.

Criterion A: The score on a standardized test of fine or gross motor co-ordination is at least 2 standard deviations below the level expected for the child's chronological age.

Criterion B: The disturbance in criterion A significantly interferes with academic achievement or with activities of daily living.

Criterion C: There is no diagnosable neurological disorder.

Criterion D: IQ is below 70 on an individually administered standardized test (most commonly used exclusion clause).

Both classifications are therefore similar and emphasize motor functions that are significantly below the level of those expected based on the child's age and intelligence and imply that DCD is therefore a specific difficulty rather than a generalized or global difficulty. These dysfunctions also significantly interfere with academic achievements and activities of daily living. However, the classifications give no indications as to possible reasons or whether there are any sub-types that need to be differentiated.

Cognition and DCD

Concerns have been raised by those working in the field of DCD regarding the use of *intelligence quotients* (IQ) as one of the criteria. In his work, Gubbay (1975) suggested that the most important single diagnostic criterion was a significantly lower performance IQ than verbal IQ (considered usually as a 15-point discrepancy on the Wechsler Intelligence Scale for Children – Revised (WISC-R)). However, the clinical experience of professionals suggests that not all children with this type of motor co-ordination dysfunction meet this criterion. Dawdy (1981) writes 'It is probably unrealistic and theoretically restrictive to assume normal or near normal intellectual capacity as a diagnostic criterion'. Needless to say, there is a general agreement that children with DCD have average intellectual capacity.

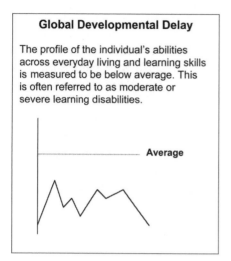

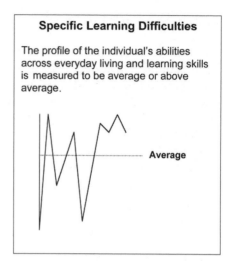

Figure 1.1 Global Developmental Delay (GDD) vs Specific Learning Difficulties (SpLD).

Aetiology

Research suggests that there is no single factor that causes DCD and that the aetiology is unclear and heterogeneous (Gubbay, 1975). Advances in studies of the brain have indicated that wide areas of the brain are involved in the planning and performance of motor actions (Rizzolatti et al., 1998; Willingham, 1998; Rowe and Frackowiak, 1999). Various causes of DCD have been investigated at different levels and a wide range of approaches has been taken to identify the source of the difficulties experienced (Barnett et al., 1998). Factors considered centred on brain damage or dysfunction, genetic predisposition, impairment in information processing or an impoverished environment. Clearly multi-causal models need to be explored (Cermak and Larkin, 2002).

Some researchers in the area of DCD have suggested that motor dysfunction in childhood may be as a result of 'minimal brain dysfunction' (Walton et al., 1962; Gubbay et al., 1965). Neurological soft signs have been examined where the researchers have found more soft signs exhibited in DCD children than in a control group. Prenatal, perinatal or postnatal incidents affecting early brain development are thought to play an important role in DCD; however, the aetiological significance for DCD remains unclear (Touwen, 1990).

Sub-types of DCD

Although the concept of children with motor co-ordination difficulties has been around for some time, it was Orton in 1937 who suggested that some children displayed varying types of problems. This was further supported by studies carried out by Walton et al. (1962) and Gubbay et al. (1965). Although these early studies and investigations were drawn from adult neurology, they set the scene for further work on sub-typing research.

Studies have generally been intent on investigating the underlying causes as if they were dealing with a unitary disorder (Smyth and Glencross, 1986; Geuze and Kalverboer, 1987; Horak et al., 1988; Murphy and Gliner, 1988; van Dellen and Geuze, 1988).

Theories postulated

- Motor planning due to sensory integration (Ayres, 1972b; Ayres et al., 1987)
- Deficits in visual perception (Gubbay, 1975; Henderson and Hall, 1982; O'Brien et al., 1988; Wilson and McKensie, 1998)
- Deficits in kinaesthetic perception (Bairstow and Laslow, 1981; Laslow and Bairstow, 1983; Wilson and McKensie, 1998)
- Deficits in timing and action (Lundy-Ekman et al., 1991; Williams et al., 1992; Piek and Skinner, 1999).

Results from studies do suggest that different sub-types of DCD exist, although it is difficult to draw comparisons and conclusions. However, some consistent patterns are becoming apparent (Cermak and Larkin, 2002).

Prevalence

Statistics of the incidence of DCD vary, but a number of studies have been undertaken and the results suggest that the incidence of DCD ranges from 3 per cent to 22 per cent of the population. The varying percentages are related to an inconsistency in definition, screening and assessment tools (Keogh et al., 1979; Losse et al., 1991; Maeland, 1992; Geuze and Borger, 1993; Revie and Larkin, 1993; Cermak and Larkin, 2002). As with many other types of developmental disability, a higher prevalence of DCD may be found in males than in females.

The incidence of DCD is found not to be related to level of education or socio-economic status (Blondis, 1999).

Table 1.1 Sub-types of DCD

Sub-type	Description of presenting features
Postural motor	Weak but normal muscle tone Trunk/girdle instability Poor grading of smoothly controlled movement Poor static and dynamic balance and quality of movement Difficulty using two sides of the body in co-ordination
Musculo-skeletal	Extreme joint laxity due to a combination of loose ligaments and low average muscle tone May adopt different compensatory postures
Neuro-motor	Minimal neurological deficits i.e. associated reactions, mirror movements, mild tightness of certain muscle groups Execution of motor acts may be affected There may be development of deviated postures
Sensory integration	Inefficiency in modulating and discriminating tactile, proprioceptive and vestibular sensory information for the development of postural motor control, perceptual processing and praxis function, thus producing an adaptive response
Perceptual motor	Poor body awareness and difficulties integrating visual and auditory information to motor output Has implications on academic learning and activities of daily living
Praxis	Primary deficits in components of praxis, namely ideation, motor planning and sequencing functions Affects the ability to learn new tasks, organize oneself across a range of living and learning skills, and be able to generalize what is learned into different situations

Source: adapted from Chu (2002).

Figures therefore indicate that DCD is a relatively common disorder and as such can be considered to be a major public health problem (Missiuna, 2001).

Children at risk

DCD is reported to be found frequently among pre-term or low birth weight children (Marlow et al., 1993; Fox and Lent, 1996). Jongmans et al. (1993,

1998), in their longitudinal study, found that some children had perceptual motor problems at school age while others did not. MRI scans indicated that some of these children presented with small lesions at birth that persisted with age. However, a study carried out by Cooke and Abernethy (1999) examined 15–17-year-old adolescents derived from a cohort of very low birth weight infants, and failed to find a relationship between lesions identified on MRI and problems with motor function. Kolb (1999) stated that there appeared to be an inconsistent relationship between motor dysfunction and underlying brain damage. However, knowledge may become clearer with the increased understanding of the interplay between neural plasticity and environmental stimulation (Kolb, 1999).

Genetic influences

Illingworth (1968), Regehr and Kaplan (1988) indicated that in some families there is evidence of a genetic influence. Gubbay (1995) noted that more often than by chance there may be a family history of motor or related neurodevelopment dysfunction. However, evidence of familial correlation derives from a variety of sources and with increasing variance.

Contributions regarding the familial theory can be found in conjunction with problems with speech and language. Studies examining dyslexia have found a behavioural phenotype with impaired motor timing (Wolff et al., 1995). Further support for heritability is evident in the study by Stordy (2000), who suggests a common basis for co-morbid dyslexia and DCD.

Current research therefore suggests that DCD is caused as a result of the interaction of the individual's make-up (genetics) and the environment (Kirby and Drew, 2002).

DCD and the differential diagnosis

It is important to point out that several of the distinguishing features of DCD are also observable in some general medical conditions. Therefore it is vital to establish the underlying cause for the motor impairment as early as possible.

Medical conditions that can mimic DCD

- cerebral palsy (CP);
- benign congenital hypotonia;
- motor disorders associated with head injury;
- global developmental delay (GDD);

- progressive muscular diseases;
- decreased motor functions related to neuro-conduction diseases, e.g. polyneuropathies;
- decreased motor functions related to seizure disorders;
- specific conditions – neurofibromatosis (NF), Ehlers Danlos (EDS); Tourette's syndrome as part of other specific developmental disorders, e.g. attention deficit and hyperactivity disorder (ADHD), Asperger's syndrome (AS).

The co-existence of DCD with other specific learning difficulties

Co-morbidity is described as a situation where two or more conditions that are diagnostically distinguishable from one another tend to occur together. However the exact nature of the relationship between co-morbid conditions is a matter still under debate (Martini et al., 1999; Clarkin and Kendall, 1992).

The evidence from recent research strongly supports the co-morbidity of the following specific learning disabilities:

- In a population study, Kaplan found that 23% of the children showed signs of DCD, 8% had features of attention deficit and hyperactivity disorder (ADHD) and 19% were seen to be dyslexic. Nearly 25% were found with ADHD, DCD and dyslexia. Only 10% had ADHD and DCD, and 22% had dyslexia and DCD only. Kaplan considers that the overlapping nature of the specific learning difficulties should lead to the use of the label of 'atypical brain disorders' rather than putting children into artificial boxes (Kaplan et al., 1998).
- Up to 52% of individuals with ADHD also have poor motor co-ordination (Hartsough and Lambert, 1985; Szatmari et al., 1989; Barkley et al., 1990).
- Up to 50% of children with DCD have moderate to severe symptoms of ADHD (Kadesjo and Gillberg, 1999).
- Individuals with Tourette's syndrome are reported to have deficits in the domains of fine motor skills, visuo-motor skills, spatial skills and executive function (Borstein, 1990; Borstein and Yang, 1991; Denckla et al., 1991).
- Rutter (1978) found that poor motor organization is prominent in autistic children.
- Wing (1981) reported motor inco-ordination to be characteristic in Asperger's syndrome. It has been included in the differential diagnosis criteria (Gillberg and Gillberg, 1989; ICD-10 (WHO, 1992).
- Individuals with specific learning difficulties (SpLD) were found to

show an increased incidence of dyspraxia (Ayres, 1972a; Cermak et al., 1980; Lennox et al. 1988; Deuel and Doar, 1992).
• Children with specific language disorders showed an increased incidence of limb dyspraxia (Aram and Horwitz, 1983; Cermak et al., 1986; Archer and Witelson, 1988; Dewey et al., 1988; Thal et al., 1991; Hill, 1998).

There is also evidence to suggest that there is co-morbidity of specific learning difficulties and other conditions that affect an individual's social, emotional, and/or behavioural functioning, such as depression, conduct disorder and oppositional/defiant disorder.

Kaplan et al. (1999) found that it was particularly difficult to determine whether one condition was in fact a symptom of the other, i.e. causality versus correlation. They further stated that these important debates aside, research evidence supports the notion that 'co-morbidity is the rule rather than the exception', and that a number of conditions co-occur with specific learning disabilities more often than would be expected 'just by chance'.

DCD is therefore considered to be a heterogeneous group with differing underlying aetiological factors. However, it is important to have an understanding and insight into the aetiology of a particular individual's clumsiness as it will help the professional to tailor an appropriate intervention strategy (Taft and Barowsky, 1989; Sellers, 1995; Willoughby and Polatajko, 1995; Smyth and Mason, 1997, 1998; Wegner, 1997; Blondis, 1999).

Presenting features and functional implications

The defining characteristic of the child and adult with DCD is one of a motor co-ordination difficulty, which may or may not be accompanied by any number of additional symptoms and overlapping disorders. The person needs to be viewed as an individual with strengths and difficulties, and consideration needs to be given to what they can and what they cannot do compared with the 'normal population'.

An individual may present with difficulties in the acquisition and mastery of any or all of the following:

• activities of daily living – dressing (buttons, sequencing and orientation of garments), feeding (using a knife and fork, food preparation), self-care (bathing, toileting, hair care);
• fine motor skills affecting manipulation of everyday tools and objects;
• gross motor skills affecting balance, co-ordination, participation in physical activities, games and leisure pursuits;
• literacy skills – spelling, reading and writing;

- numeracy skills – sequencing of numbers;
- self and work organization;
- attention and concentration;
- social skills.

Secondary implications

- difficulty making and maintaining friendships/relationships;
- negative behaviour;
- low self-esteem and confidence;
- anxiety.

The characteristics and developmental course of DCD will be discussed in the next chapter and will form the basis for the information-gathering process relating to assessment in Chapter 4.

Summary

Research suggests that individuals with poor co-ordination have been around for a long time, where the incidence ranges from 3 per cent to 22 per cent of the population, with more males being affected than females. The evidence from recent research strongly supports the view that DCD co-exists with other specific learning difficulties.

There is no single factor that causes DCD. It is heterogeneous and its aetiology remains unclear.

Although research to date has only begun to explore the underlying mechanism, there is a growing consensus that the multi-dimensional nature of DCD cannot be explained by single factors. As with many other developmental conditions, the long-term consequences are much more likely to arise from multiple interacting factors, and cannot be understood in isolation from the normal age-related developmental processes. Neurodevelopment, cognitive, environmental and experiential processes all play an important part in shaping the individual.

There remains an inconsistency in the term used to define this disorder, despite an international consensus. Further, frequent changes in the name of the condition reflect the fact that the underlying aetiology for DCD is still not yet fully understood.

However, what is known is that DCD is not a disease and it cannot be transmitted. Neither is it life threatening. There are no blood tests for it like those for arthritis, heart disease and diabetes. It cannot be cured; neither surgery nor drugs have anything to offer (Fox, 1998).

It is therefore important to view the emergence and development of the concept of DCD as a *dynamic process* (Henderson and Barnett, 1998).

CHAPTER 2

The developmental course of DCD

Until recently, problems with motor co-ordination in childhood were thought to be of minor importance, typically outgrown in adolescence or adulthood.

A number of studies have examined the movement skills problems of school-age children and tried to determine whether the problems persist over time or whether the children 'grow out of them'. Losse et al. (1991) report on four of these studies and conclude that it is 'erroneous to believe that children with mild to moderate motor difficulties grow out of them'.

Research suggests that for individuals with mild to moderate DCD, the outcome into adulthood is good, as many individuals will probably learn to compensate for their difficulties. Some individuals seem to benefit from their growth spurt, which may have been caused by enhancement in the maturation of parts of their Central Nervous System (CNS) (Visser et al., 1998).

Furthermore, studies indicate that at least 50 per cent of motor-impaired children will still have motor difficulties as adults, and many of them will develop secondary difficulties in the areas of physical health, mental health, social well-being, and educational performance and achievements. Many will be unfit and have poor social competence, academic problems, behavioural problems, and low self-esteem (Shafer et al., 1986; Gillberg and Gillberg, 1989; Gillberg et al., 1989; Losse et al., 1991; Geuze and Borger, 1993; Hellgren et al., 1993; Cantell et al., 1994; Schoemaker and Kalverboer, 1994; Bouffard et al., 1996).

The significance of early developmental history

Gubbay (1978, 1985) investigated birth histories of children with DCD and reported a significant history of prenatal, perinatal or neonatal factors in 50 per cent of the cases. He also noted a higher ratio of first-born children. However, as only half of those studied presented with histories, the findings were not significant enough to be able to relate the birth history to the incidence of DCD.

DCD in its milder forms will not be detected during the first few years of life as the child usually achieves motor milestones within normal limits, albeit often slowly (Gubbay, 1985).

Pre-school

At this age, the child may present with high activity levels and awkward movement skills, both at a gross and fine motor level. Their play skills may lack imagination and creativity. Their language appears to be fine, as the child is only using high frequency words.

It may not be easy to identify any major difficulties with the child's performance, and their ability may be seen as reasonably consistent with their peers. Any gap may not be that great, and expectations not so high. In addition, as the child is more likely to be male, it may be assumed that any delay in his mastery of everyday living and learning skills is due to his sex, i.e. it is generally accepted that boys develop at a slower rate than girls at this stage.

Observable characteristics

- Persistent feeding difficulties – intolerance, restricted diet;
- Evidence of sleeping difficulties – poor bedtime routines, constant waking requiring reassurance;
- Uncoordinated movement – unsteady when walking, unable to pedal a tricycle;
- Difficulties with fine motor skills – avoids pencil activities, and manipulating small objects in play;
- High levels of motor activity – constantly on the go;
- Insecurity – separating from adult;
- High levels of excitability;
- Toilet training may be delayed;
- Delayed language development;
- Concentration limited compared to peers;
- Lack of imaginative play;
- Unresolved hand preference;
- Peer isolation;
- Sensitive to sensory stimulation;
- Limited response to verbal instructions – sequencing, slowness in processing.

The primary years

Current practices in primary education are now making greater demands on children's co-ordination and the amount of time devoted to developing prerequisite movement skills is decreasing. The teacher education structure also does not provide adequately for them to feel confident and competent in the area of children's movement development skills. The more active the school curriculum becomes, the more some of the children with inefficient motor performance will have negative experiences in a greater range of school subjects (Stafford, 2000).

At this stage the children begin to develop insight. They find it difficult to make sense of what is going on around them. Learning new skills is difficult and they do not know why. Behavioural manifestations such as temper tantrums and acting out may become apparent.

In school, the environment becomes more structured. Activities that could have been avoided without notice on the playground or in a nursery setting now have to be confronted head-on as they are integral to the curriculum. Here the child has to handle and deal with increasing amounts of information and demands upon their sensory motor skills (Kirby and Drew, 2002).

Deficits in play skills become more evident, and studies by Primeau (1992) and Bouffard et al. (1996) demonstrated that children with DCD were less likely to be vigorously active or play on large equipment. Further, there is a body of research that suggests that the DCD child tends to be more passive in play and more anxious than other children. Bundy (2002) suggests that children with DCD are likely to be less competent and therefore less accepted by their peers, leading to isolation and reinforced feelings of low self-worth.

This is further supported by Wetton (1997), who observed that children who are 'clumsy' or socially inept are not tolerated by their peers if they show any deviation from expected playing styles. Yet other children who have more visible 'special needs' are accepted.

Observable characteristics
- organizational difficulties emerging;
- difficulties adapting to routines;
- difficulties in PE and games;
- difficulties with personal care – dressing;
- literacy difficulties emerge – spelling, writing (pencil control);
- numeracy difficulties emerge;
- deficits in attention and concentration;
- highly emotional;

- difficulty with social relationships;
- avoidance behaviours;
- perceived as immature compared to peers;
- difficulty following and interpreting verbal information.

The middle school years

In the middle school years there is a dramatic increase in the demands for written output (Levine, 1987). Geuze and Borger (1993) suggest that children with DCD are more likely to be held back a year or be placed in lower sets in school. The extent to which the school environment influences success or failure has also been commented upon. Despite new legislation, directives and policy, it still appears that some schools are better than others at maximizing the learning capabilities of their pupils (Stafford, 2000).

In her study, Levine (1984) concluded that 'being bright helped to compensate for the problem, but did not make the child feel any better'. Failure to keep up with work was more likely to result in a decline in grades and in motivation and self-esteem. Children with DCD frequently become the victims of bullying which creates further distress (Portwood, 2000).

A child's retrospective view

At the age of 10 I was referred by my doctor to a child psychiatrist. All I remember was I felt an overwhelming feeling of being 'on trial'. I felt he was questioning my sanity rather than addressing the difficulties I was facing.

My school years were a blur of underachievement and loneliness. I had no close friends and significantly at any time no girlfriend. (Amory)

Observable characteristics
- organizational difficulties of self and work;
- forgetful – no sense of time;
- continued difficulties in PE and games;
- can usually dress but still has problems with orientation of garments, fastenings and shoelaces;
- literacy difficulties – spelling, writing – content, organization, presentation and speed;
- numeracy problems;
- attention and concentration difficulties;
- difficulties with social relationships;
- avoidance behaviours – may be class clown or disruptive;
- perceived as immature compared to peers;
- difficulty following and interpreting verbal information.

Adolescents and adulthood

In secondary school, fast handwriting, keyboard skills, organization, social skills and games become more important (Stafford, 2000).

In their study, Losse et al. (1991) found that at the age of 16 the children continued to experience substantial motor difficulties as well as a variety of educational, social and emotional problems. Academically they were considered to be less successful than their peers despite similar effort. They were also more likely to have lower academic ambitions and a poorer self-concept than their peers. This, it was reported, is likely to affect the type of career choices the individual makes, as he perceives himself to be less able than he may actually be.

Parent feedback in this study also suggested that the schools' lack of concern about the child's motor difficulties was a major determinant of behaviour problems. The study also highlighted that, in some cases, the academic and social demands of being in a large school had not only increased their existing difficulties but also revealed new ones.

In their study, Skinner and Piek (2001) suggested that individuals with DCD were found to perceive themselves as less competent in several areas and received less social support. Further, they found that overall the adolescents had lower self-worth and higher levels of anxiety. The longer-term implications of anxiety potentially led to an increased risk of depression in adulthood (Fox and Lent, 1996).

While there has been a marked increase in the awareness of DCD, it appears that the knowledge base is greater within the primary setting, rather than the secondary. A comparison of features between childhood and adulthood is illustrated in Table 2.1.

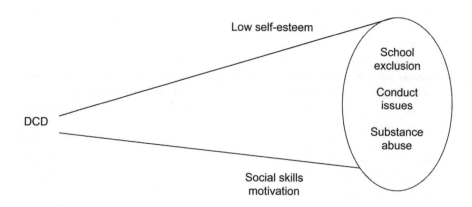

Figure 2.1 Unmanaged DCD.

Table 2.1 Comparison of features – childhood vs adulthood

PHYSICAL

Issue	Childhood	Adulthood
Co-ordination of limbs	Hopping Skipping Playground games and PE Riding a bike Ball skills Dressing Personal care	Avoid leisure activities – ball sports, cycling Domestic tasks Driving car, motor bike Personal care Operation of equipment and machinery
Flexibility and range of motion – stiffness, fitness	Fitness, endurance, stamina (for school) – health Sitting, standing posture Leisure activities – ball sports, cycling	Fitness, endurance, stamina (for college, university, work) – health Sitting, standing posture Leisure activities – ball sports, cycling
Dexterity Poorly established hand preference, immature grips	Grips and grasps for picking up and holding tools – writing, scissors, pencils, brushes Personal care – buttons and fastenings Using cutlery and eating	Quality of writing Operation of equipment and machinery – work and home Assembly of objects – work and home Personal care – buttons and fastenings Using kitchen utensils, knives, opening jars, scissors
Eye/hand co-ordination Visual tracking	Ball games Copying from the board Cutting with scissors	Sports Cooking/domestic skills Work skills – filing

EXECUTIVE FUNCTION

Issue	Childhood	Adulthood
Problem-solving, organization of self and belongings	Study skills Planning and organization of self and time and belongings in the classroom Writing Sequencing Play Games and PE	Study skills Planning and organization of self and time and belongings Sequencing of tasks and prioritizing Writing Workplace Leisure Home Management/organization Orienteering Managing appointments

Table 2.1 continued

EXECUTIVE FUNCTION

Issue	Childhood	Adulthood
Learning styles – literacy and numeracy	Study skills – meeting National Curriculum targets Telling time Memory retrieval – information	Unfinished school/ education/ under-achieved academically Study skills Keeping up-to-date with news Interpreting information – bills, circulars, legal information Managing finances Telling time Form completion Memory retrieval for information Work issues – multiple jobs, problems with authority, colleagues
Attention and concentration	Listen in class Follow instructions from teacher/parent Task completion – shift attention from one thing to another Filter out extraneous noise and visual stimuli	Listen to others – work/home Task completion – shift attention from one thing to another Filter out extraneous noise and visual stimuli Safety – driving, operating machinery/equipment

DAILY LIVING

Issue	Childhood	Adulthood
Social skills	Making and keeping friends Understanding social rules Understanding rules of play and games Coping with change and uncertainty Interpreting pragmatic language (facial expression, gesture, tone of voice)	Making and keeping friends Understanding social rules Coping with change and uncertainty Poor relationships – multiple relationships Interpreting pragmatic language (facial expression, gesture, tone of voice)
Community living skills	Accessing clubs and out-of-school activities Road safety Finding way around local area Using public transport and public amenities Using local shops	Accessing clubs, pubs, restaurants Road safety Finding way around local area and wider geographical area Using public transport (trains, planes) and public amenities Using wide range of retail outlets

Table 2.1 continued

DAILY LIVING

Issue	Childhood	Adulthood
Survival skills and activities of daily living	What to do if lost What to do in an emergency – who to contact in case of fire, emergency Basic first aid Make self snack, drink Using phone Personal care Reading community and social signs	What to do in an emergency Basic first aid Catering for self and others/family/pets Caring for health needs and managing medication Domestic skills Home maintenance Reading community and social signs Orienteering

PSYCHOLOGICAL WELL-BEING/ HEALTH

Issue	Childhood	Adulthood
Emotional health, self-perception	Motivation – taking risks Accepting of strengths, differences and needs Self-esteem, confidence Self-acceptance Body image Emotional regulation Environmental and emotional sensitivity Life roles – son/daughter, friend, pupil	Motivation – taking risks Accepting of strengths, differences and needs Self-esteem and confidence Self-acceptance Body image Managing stress Emotional regulation Environmental and emotional sensitivity Dietary issues and weight gain Life roles – husband/wife, employee, mother/father

Looking back at his school days, one adult with DCD wrote:

If there is anything I've learnt from my life, it's that DCD has to be viewed in its entirety. Worrying about school to the exclusion of everything else may produce an academically very capable adult who will still be unable to cope, as the lack of confidence, speech problems and social difficulties remain unresolved. (Werenowska, 2003, p. 16)

Cantell's study (1998) reported that adolescents with DCD were less sociable and more passive, with their behaviour being described as 'socially negative'. This supported Geuze and Borger's study (1993), which found that adolescents with DCD had less developed social contacts and friendships. In contrast to these findings, which appear to show a passive (internalizing) behavioural pattern, Losse et al. (1991) found behavioural patterns which varied from bullying to police offences (Cermak and Larkin, 2002).

In terms of engagement in activities such as hobbies and leisure pursuits, Cantell et al. (1994) found that the individual with DCD engaged in fewer hobbies. Larkin and Parker (1999) found that playing computer games was more common in the DCD group.

With regard to employment, Knuckey and Gubbay (1983) found that adolescents with extreme motor problems had the least skilled jobs. This was further supported by Losse et al. (1991), who reported that by the age of 16, adolescents diagnosed with DCD at 6 years of age not only had lower school achievement, but as a consequence, some of them found it hard to gain employment (Cantell, 1998). On a positive note, many adults with DCD develop adaptive characteristics and achieve goals by unconventional means, devise different ways of doing things, or avoid them.

It appears that a combination of personal and environmental factors plays an aggravating role in the adolescent educational/academic outcome of DCD. While studies suggest that adults with DCD continue to have experience of motor control difficulties, the secondary manifestations of the disorder now emerge as the primary features (see Figure 2.2). This is a key factor in the identification and assessment process, as the type of service that the adult may enter as a result, e.g. mental health services, is potentially unlikely to explore the developmental background of the individual.

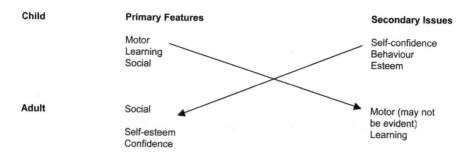

Figure 2.2 Primary features/secondary issues – the interchange.

Observable characteristics – adolescents
- difficulties with social relationships/friendships;
- difficulties with organization – homework, timetables, task completion;

- low productivity – slow to complete work/tasks;
- emotional/behavioural issues;
- problems with motor co-ordination;
- difficulty with recording of information – speed, organization, presentation;
- short-term auditory and visual memory difficulties;
- easily led;
- obsessional behaviours;
- immature compared with peers;
- difficulties with self-care and personal independence skills.

Observable characteristics – adults
- obsessional characteristics;
- co-ordination difficulties – affecting home maintenance, learning to drive;
- poor handwriting;
- low self-esteem;
- emotional problems;
- unrealistic expectations;
- difficulty remembering instructions;
- organizational difficulties – home management/work;
- inability to complete tasks quickly;
- difficulties with job retention;
- difficulty making decisions;
- depression;
- difficulty maintaining relationships/partnerships;
- sleeping difficulties;
- high co-morbidity with ADHD and psychiatric illness.

Adults with DCD – their points of view

An extract from Ceri's story

From beginning to end, my life has been one long struggle, but very early on I decided that I could either laugh or cry at my difficulties and I fortunately decided to laugh. I do try to think positively about all the things I can do, rather than those I can't, but sometimes I feel that having DCD is a bit like starting out on a big, noisy motorway. At the beginning everyone seems to be going in the same direction, but for some reason those with DCD don't seem to understand the signposts and then suddenly lots of obstacles appear. This means that we have to stop and take a detour, hoping that we will catch up with the others later. Somehow I never seem to have got back on to the motorway, instead I have gone on B roads and ended up in a village with no way out. I feel that I need some help to get over the obstacles ahead of me in the hope that I might one day get to where I really want to go – the big city of Employment. (Werenowska, 2003, p. 26)

Much literature focuses on the deficits of DCD rather than the positives. Adults with DCD are now keen that their voice is heard promoting the strengths of DCD. One organization (Dyspraxia Adults Action) lists the following strengths:

Adults with DCD

- are able to learn with determination and plenty of practice;
- can be creative and original thinkers;
- have a good sense of humour which they use at times to get them through adversity;
- are fond of and good at caring for animals, as pets give unconditional love and do not judge them by their appearance or ability;
- have empathy for others and often are successful in professions such as caring or teaching;
- are hard-working and determined to succeed;
- are honest, genuine and sincere, because they do not put on a false act to impress others.

Table 2.2 Focus on strengths not weaknesses

Weakness	Strength
Hyperactivity	Energy to work and play
Hyper-focusing	Concentration needed to organize self
Distractible	Keeping an eye on what's going on
Slow	Or is it methodical? Make fewer mistakes More disciplined approach
Perceptual problems and disorganized thinking	Have a creative approach Thinking is helpful for fresh viewpoints
Overcompensate	Listen well Or look for detail
Don't pay attention to detail	See the bigger picture
Poor literacy and numeracy	Better developed verbal skills
Experiences of rejection	Determined

They are also described as:

- being creative problem-solvers, as the individual needs to work around their disability; this allows them to think 'outside the box', often leading to more creative solutions and imaginative answers to problems;
- being outgoing personalities – many develop this in an attempt to compensate for their difficulties;
- having strong compensatory skills;
- being persistent – despite frustrations, many keep trying until they meet with success (National Adult Literacy and Learning Disabilities, 1999).

Summary

Longitudinal studies on DCD have attempted to consider whether DCD is a temporary or a persisting disorder (Cermak and Larkin, 2002). The current picture that is emerging is that some children with minor problems in childhood seem to 'grow out of it'. However, the more severely affected children remain 'clumsy' and are at risk of developing associated problems.

The manifestations of this disorder therefore vary with age and development. Poor motor performance is often found alongside academic performance deficits. In primary school, actions such as constructing, writing, drawing, playing are all part of everyday school life; in secondary school, fast handwriting, keyboard skills, organization, social skills and games become more important. At home, personal care and domestic skills are essential prerequisites to independent living. In adulthood, the individual often continues to have difficulty with recording information, organization, time management and social interaction.

Table 2.3 Summary of factors affecting the outlook for individuals with DCD

Supporting factors	Hindering factors
Milder core symptoms	Severe core symptoms
Early diagnosis	Late diagnosis/no diagnosis
High IQ	Low average IQ
Limited overlapping features	High proportion of overlapping features
Good family relationships	Poor family relationships
Supportive extended family/access to community activities	Isolation from family and community
Educational/work environment co-operative and supportive	Educational/work environment unco-operative and unsupportive

To date, the question as to why some individuals with DCD improve and others do not is unresolved. However, as with many other developmental disorders, the long-term behavioural consequences of DCD are likely to arise from multiple interacting factors and cannot be understood in isolation from normal age-related developmental processes (Cermak and Larkin, 2002). Therefore, it is essential to have an understanding and an insight into these dynamics and sequences of the processes in order to understand and prepare appropriately for the outcome i.e. service provision.

CHAPTER 3

Assessment

Diagnostic labels in adults – help or hindrance?

The presenting features of DCD are not visible as are other conditions such as cerebral palsy. Many individuals refer to themselves as having a hidden handicap. It is easy to recognize severe dysfunction because the individual is observably or catastrophically unable to perform everyday living and learning tasks. It is much harder to recognize, prevent or remediate the impending onset of dysfunction or performance deficits, which, although they do not result in total inability, are nevertheless subtly and cumulatively damaging to the life of the individual. This is the case for DCD.

Conditions such as DCD can feed upon themselves and lead to a downward spiral. They not only dis-enable the individual but also disempower them. However, if an individual is able to recognize this, seek help and use help, the need for prolonged intervention is lessened. However, a paradox exists that those most likely to need assistance are also those who are less likely to be able to seek and make use of it (Hagadorn, 2001).

It is widely accepted that perceptions of dysfunction are culturally loaded (Hagedorn, 2001), where it can be difficult to draw the line between those who are genuinely dysfunctional, and those whom society labels as 'odd' or 'deviant' because they do not conform to the social norms of the majority. It is therefore important not to use 'labels' that are associated with dysfunction too loosely.

A label can be seen to be both positive and negative. It can:

- acknowledge to the individual that their worries and concerns are valid and confirmation of DCD can allow them to 'make sense' of their past and move on;
- enable the individual to access financial help or services;
- be used as an excuse: 'I can't because I have DCD', or be seen as a 'middle-class' excuse for the individual not doing as well academically;
- assist with research, e.g. causation, intervention and for planning future services;

- be seen as a 'life sentence', i.e. individuals see themselves as disabled rather than able with difficulties that can improved or managed.

However, seeking help as an adult has been found to be difficult. Many will have known all of their life that something was 'different about them'. They have read an article in the paper or seen a feature on TV. Some still live with parents who continue to seek help on their behalf. As many have emotional difficulties or musculo-skeletal difficulties (back pain, pain on walking), they may enter services that are not aware of DCD. This perceived lack of remedy for their symptoms, and not knowing where to go to get help, may cause individuals to move from one service to another seeking help. This can potentially lead individuals to gain a reputation for being a 'hypochondriac' or a 'nuisance'. Many are driven to alternative services. In the UK the Adult Dyspraxia Group now provides valuable support and signposting.

> I was so relieved to finally understand my problems and to be able to explain what was causing them to other people. It helped take away a sense of shame I'd been living with for all these years. Having a diagnosis helped me work around my limitations. Having it all out in the open has relieved me of most of my anxiety and I no longer take antidepressants'. (Adult with DCD)

Nevertheless, the increasing awareness of DCD in children is beginning to have a follow-through into the education system and beyond, with special needs co-ordinators and advisory teachers being key in identification and remediation. Within further and higher education, disability officers are becoming more aware and can enable students to access help. Furthermore, policy and directives from Government relating to disability have also now made employers more aware of hidden disabilities such as

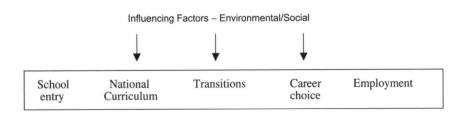

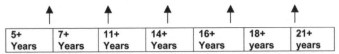

Figure 3.1 Milestone trigger points for accessing services.

DCD and related conditions. It is now possible for employees to access disability employment advisers (DEAs) for support within the workplace.

Figure 3.1 illustrates potential trigger points for individuals with DCD to access services. Figures 3.2 and 3.3 illustrate the differing referral pathways for the child compared with the adult.

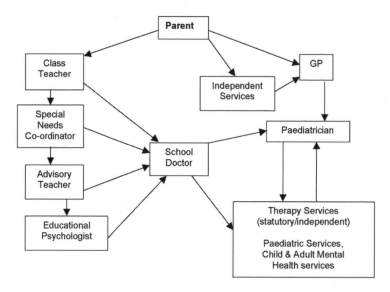

Figure 3.2 Child schema – referral pathways.

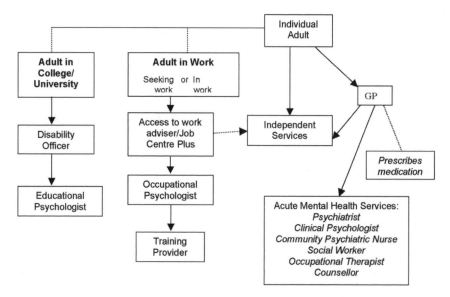

Figure 3.3 Adult schema – referral pathways.

Assessment of DCD

As discussed in previous chapters, there is little in terms of literature available regarding adolescents and adults with DCD. It is therefore necessary to return once more to studies on children to construct the way forward.

Longitudinal studies are at present hampered by several factors, namely poor screening criteria, and the heterogeneity of the movement difficulties (Cermak and Larkin, 2002). Further, the diagnostic criteria for developmental disorders in the DSM IV do not take into account the possible change in the manifestation of the disorder with age. Figure 3.4 illustrates the co-existence of features which impact on the assessment process.

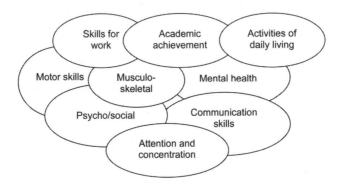

Figure 3.4 Co-existence of features in adults which influence assessment.

Features that may initially present in adults

- mental health problems – anxiety, depression, obsessional traits;
- physical manifestations – back, hip, neck, knee pain, pain on walking;
- difficulties with job retention and employability – workplace issues:
- academic problems.

Issues around existing assessment methods

Neurodevelopmental

Studies have concentrated on changes in the occurrence of 'soft' signs on clinical examination, e.g. Touwen's (1979) Examination. Although some children with soft signs may have been diagnosed with DCD, others have been found to move competently. In general, puberty is related to a decrease in soft neurological signs (Gillberg et al., 1989; Soorani-Lunsing et al., 1993).

Descriptive motor tests

These include measures such as the Movement ABC Battery (Henderson and Sugden, 1992) and the Bruininks-Oseretsky (Bruininks, 1978), and are aimed at assessing functional performance in everyday actions using chronological age against which performance is judged. Although these descriptor tests have been developed to assess motor performance during primary and middle school, so far well-standardized motor tests for older populations are limited (Losse et al., 1991).

Interviews

These have been used in studies with DCD. However, they have mainly concentrated on either psychiatric symptoms (Shafer et al., 1986; Hellgren et al., 1994) or on personal interests (Losse et al., 1991; Cantell et al., 1994) and provide a more qualitative picture.

Observation

This is core to assessment; it is the process by which observers use operation definitions as a guide. Longitudinal studies using this method have not yet been done. Although observational scales for motor testing do exist (Kalverboer et al., 1990; Henderson and Sugden, 1992), there is a need for observational scales specifically designed for everyday activities in adolescents and adults with DCD.

Assessment context

Research suggests that there is no one gold standard assessment; it is recommended that evaluation should be multi-dimensional and that

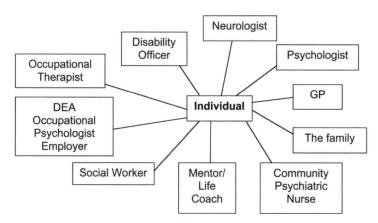

Figure 3.5 The team.

evaluation should take place over a period of time and different contexts i.e. work, home, learning, environment and community.

In view of the high levels of co-morbidity, any number of professionals have the potential to become involved with an adult with DCD. Figure 3.5 identifies key team members and the role they can play in the assessment/intervention of an adult with DCD.

Methods of assessment

Generally the term 'assessment' is used to describe such actions as examining, measuring, testing or observing an individual using structured formats, and comparing observed performance to specified criteria, standards and norms. The aims of assessment are summarized below in Table 3.1.

Table 3.1 Aims of assessment

To diagnose	To discover the nature of the problem, condition or situation To identify areas of strength and weakness, noting areas of dysfunction within everyday living and learning skills
To explore subjective responses	Individual's perception concerns and responses
To evaluate • To set a baseline • To measure • To chart progress	In order to plan intervention/remediation or to quantify change Specific physical capacity level of skill or ability To measure by objective means whether improvement has been made
To quantify learning	To see if learning/skill acquisition has taken place effectively
To reassure concerning progress	To illustrate progress for the individual
To provide outcome data	Assessment results may be used for managerial processes regarding service provision
To predict: • To plan future action • To enable individual to make decisions • To inform co-professionals	Need for further intervention Concerns personal future and actions So individual can include information in own decision-making

Source: adapted from Hagedorn (2001).

Assessment may be:

- descriptive – stating an objective view of a person usually in comparison to some pre-determined norm, scale or standard; this is usually the most simple of the forms of assessment since it requires accurate observation, measurement and recording on only one occasion;
- evaluative – noting the changes in an individual over time; this is more complex and implies a higher degree of reliability and validity if results are to be meaningfully compared;
- predictive – making a statement about how, in consequence, the individual will be in a given situation at some future point in time; this is based on probabilities.

Testing

This may comprise the following:

- *Standardized* – These have a set procedure and results which can be compared with and rated against normative scores obtained by testing a sufficient, selected sample of people. If validated the procedure has been tested to ensure results are consistent in use.
- *Non-standardized* – These are not related to normative scores or tested for validity or inter-rated reliability. A 'criterion' is a referenced assessment of which some individual performance or goal given as a baseline is the most useful non-standardized test.

Assessment may be:

- *Informal*: Observations made in a natural setting.

Forms of observation (Polgar and Thomas, 1991)

Non-participant	'Fly on the wall'
The complete observer	One who neither interacts with the individual nor discloses his purpose
Participant observation	The observer takes part in the situation being studied
The complete participator	One who is totally immersed and becomes part of the situation
The participant as an observer	One who participates fully but discloses his identity as an observer

- *Formal*: Happening at one particular time in predetermined circumstances for a specific purpose and recorded in a precise and structured manner.

Interview – taking a history

Interviews as a research tool can offer a reflection of the everyday life and the self-understanding of an individual with DCD. They can capture 'real' examples describing the experiential world of the individual (Mulderij, 1996). They can reveal important information not found through questionnaires or formal testing.

Interviews should take the form of establishing a well-documented history through the knowledge and understanding of normal development and the range of specific learning difficulties. The interview should also encompass education and social background. Information can be gathered by using history interview forms, pre-assessment questionnaires sent out before the appointment. Ideally the interviewer should have previously obtained or had access to any previous reports from other professionals, as well as results from any previous investigations carried out (school/college, therapy).

A history elicited from the parent, if possible, and the individual, is likely to be much more eloquent than the most comprehensive examination. There will probably be evidence of delay in acquiring a number of skills through childhood, such as the ability to dress independently, feeding – using cutlery, personal care skills, pre-writing, use of tools, kicking and catching a ball, running, pedalling a bike. However, it should be remembered that all skills are influenced by cultural and family expectations, and although norms for all these milestones are available, there is wide individual variation. Clumsiness may be generalized, restricted to groups of somewhat similar tasks or highly task-specific. It is the extreme difficulty and distress experienced in trying to master one or more of these skills that distinguishes them from their peers. Even if the task is learnt it tends to be performed very slowly and inconsistently. It is important for the professional to listen to the individual and family members (if appropriate) to elicit the clues, hours spent daily unsuccessfully trying to learn simple tasks, emotional outbursts evoked by simple activities that others would find easy, the bright articulate individual failing to complete work or being totally disorganized.

History taking should consider:

- past and present symptoms;
- psychiatric history and prescribed medications;
- educational, social and employment histories;
- information regarding the individual's general ability to meet the demands of daily life.

An example of a screening checklist and history information summary is illustrated in Figure 3.6.

FUNCTIONAL AREA	YES	NO	COMMENTS
Planning and movement (gross motor skills) ➢ Clumsy gait and movement in general, difficulty changing direction, stopping and starting. Poor quality of movement and control of movement ➢ Poor posture – weak muscle tone and strength, reduced stamina Difficulty standing for long periods ➢ Overflow and exaggerated accessory movements ➢ Lack of body awareness in space ➢ Lack of rhythm ➢ Possibly late reaching infant motor milestones – walking, talking, sitting and standing ➢ Tendency to bump into other people, bump into things and trip over ➢ Difficulty in mastering childhood functional skills – riding a bike learning to dress – managing buttons ➢ Driving a car ➢ Difficulty with sports, ball games and team games ➢ Lack of rhythm – dancing, playing instruments, aerobics			
Eye/hand co-ordination ➢ Manual dexterity – unscrewing things, sewing, managing locks with keys, craft work, mechanical things, domestic chores, DIY ➢ Handwriting – pen grip, may not always finish work, press too hard, too soft ➢ Personal care – make-up, doing hair, tendency to look untidy, shaving			
Perception ➢ Difficulty translating messages into actions ➢ Following instructions – not instinctive, needs to be taught step by step ➢ Little sense of time, direction, speed, weight – poor map-reading, confusion over hand preference, left/right discrimination ➢ Difficulty distinguishing sounds/screening them from background noise. Can be over-sensitive to noise			
Language ➢ Continuous talking ➢ Understanding and using complex verbal and written language ➢ Understanding and using para-linguistic features (volume, intonation, pitch, rate, fluency, nasality, vocal quality) ➢ Understanding and using non-verbal communication (posture, facial expression) ➢ Eye contact, gesture, touch, proximity, sounds – groans, sighs, 'tuts' ➢ Pragmatic social communication (initiation, turn-taking) ➢ Perspective taking, topic selection and maintenance, clarification and repair, compromise, negotiation, accepting and giving criticism (appropriate style to situation)			
Thought and memory ➢ Difficulty planning and organizing thoughts ➢ Unfocused, messy, cluttered, erratic ➢ Poor memory (especially short-term) and may keep forgetting and losing ➢ May find it hard to do more than one thing at once ➢ Slow to finish tasks if finished at all ➢ May daydream and wander about aimlessly ➢ May have literacy and numeracy difficulties			

Figure 3.6 Adult DCD Screening Checklist.

Social and emotional problems ➤ Tendency to be easily frustrated – have emotional outbursts and be impulsive ➤ Difficulties with listening – especially in large groups ➤ May find it difficult picking up on non-verbal signals and judging the tone or pitch of voice in themselves and others. Wants immediate satisfaction ➤ Can play the clown ➤ Can be slow to adapt to new situations and learn new skills ➤ Can have problems with teamwork and have a tendency to take evasive action when they face a difficult situation ➤ May be insomniac, stressed, depressed, anxious and indecisive ➤ May have phobias, fears and obsessions ➤ May have lack of self-esteem and difficulties being assertive ➤ Tendency to opt out of things that may be too difficult ➤ Prone to emotional outbursts			

Figure 3.6 Adult DCD Screening Checklist (contd).

Personal Details – name, age, address Medical History – medication, surgery Family History – any other family members with a specific learning difficulty Early Developmental History – milestones School History – Primary/Secondary Further Education/University Work History – job retention Social History – relationships, friendships, history of bullying Previous Assessments – when and with whom (copies if possible) Current Functional Difficulties – everyday skills, work skills, social skills Concerns and Expectations Tests to be Carried Out

Figure 3.7 Adult History Information Summary.

Medical assessment

The traditional neurological examination is largely unhelpful and any abnormalities seen are not usually associated with DCD and may suggest further investigation or consultation. The nature of qualitative differences changes over time as the demands in adulthood differ from those in childhood; however, minor motor impairments are likely to be detectable in individuals with DCD as they get older. Some of these motor differences can be objectively quantified, including timing and accuracy of movements (Fox, 1998).

General medical conditions may contribute to clumsiness. These may include hearing loss, visual impairment, the effects of drugs and toxic substances, thyroid malfunction etc.

Comprehensive diagnosis should include a search for co-morbidities, particularly mood, attentional, behaviour and learning disorders that may benefit from specific interventions.

DCD is not thought to have focal brain abnormalities, and studies such as magnetic resonance imaging (MRI) and computed tomography (CT) are not useful in evaluation (Wegner, 1997).

Table 3.2 illustrates certain neuro-developmental tests which have been used, and certainly in children these have been found to be commonly

Table 3.2 Gross motor tasks and underlying neurological functions

Test	Description	Abnormal result	Neuro-developmental skill tested
Rapid alternating movement	Individual quickly alternates pronation and supination of the hand	Dysdiadochokinesis (excessive flailing)	Requires ability to inhibit proximal muscle groups
Sustained motor stance	Stand erect for 15 seconds with arms extended, feet together	Inability to maintain position	Balance, somaesthetic input, vestibular function
Tandem balance	Individual stands with one foot directly in front of the other, holding posture for 15 seconds with eyes closed	Inability to sustain posture	Motor monitoring, self-righting skills, vestibular function, somaesthetic input, balance, body position sense, selective motor inhibition, motor persistence
Hopping in place	Individual hops in place alternating between left and right foot in a specified sequence	Inability to hop, inability to perform particular hopping pattern, poor rhythm	Motor planning, motor sequencing, short-term memory, ability to set and maintain rhythm

Source: Levine (1996).

abnormal. Usefulness in adults is to be determined; however, they are helpful in the evaluation process in excluding any neurological problems and eliminate any other potential diagnosis.

Differential diagnosis in the adult

As with children with DCD, the distinguishable features in adults are also observable in some general medical and psychological/psychiatric conditions. Therefore it is vital to establish the underlying cause as promptly as possible and eliminate any other potential diagnoses.

Table 3.3 Differential diagnosis by history and physical findings

Findings	Differential diagnosis
Loss of skills	Degenerative disorders
Ataxia, dysarthria, dysmetria	Cerebellar damage
Poor muscle tone	Peripheral nerve disease
Increased muscle tone	Cerebral palsy
Asymmetry of muscle tone	Cortical damage on side of brain or spinal cord
Absent deep tendon reflexes	Muscular or peripheral nerve disease
Hyperpigmented macules	Neurofibromatosis
Skeletal abnormalities	Orthopaedic disorders, genetic disorders
Dysmorphic faces, minor physical abnormalities (ear length, hand, finger lengths)	Genetic syndrome

Other considerations: generalized learning difficulties, ADHD, acquired brain injury, mental health issues such as depression

Source: adapted from Hamilton (2002).

Assessment tools

Areas of assessment in adulthood

- Physical/motor skills – musculo-skeletal, neurological and functional
- Work skills organization, executive skills/problem-solving skills, sequencing, structured/unstructured environments
- Independent living skills
- Sensory skills – visual/perceptual, auditory, tactile
- Cognitive – short/long-term memory, attention/concentration, orientation to time, place, person (temporal), directions for performance –

writing, verbal, reading, abstract thinking, the use of already known information or provision of opportunities to learn experience by trial and error
- Psychological factors – insight, self-esteem, confidence, motivation
- Social and interpersonal skills – verbal/non-verbal skills

Table 3.4 lists tests available and considered appropriate in the information-gathering process for adults with DCD. Details of suppliers and authors can be found in Appendix IX.

Physical testing

Individuals with DCD commonly have low muscle strength (Casperson et al., 1985). Poor muscle strength in the trunk (body) may indicate a potential to develop musculo-skeletal problems. Assessment can be through:

- assessing strength and endurance – push-ups, pull-ups, bench stepping, sit-ups, grip strength;
- cardiovascular endurance runs.

Flexibility, the range of motion through which joints are able to move, varies markedly in DCD and may vary from joint to joint or between sides. Lack of flexibility can contribute to injury and long-term musculo-skeletal problems, whereas flexibility can result in joint instability and potential strain on muscles or dislocated joints. Within the DCD population extreme ranges of flexibility can be observed (Cermak and Larkin, 2002).

Coming to terms with a diagnosis

Correct identification of DCD in itself constitutes an invaluable intervention. The longstanding anxiety that 'something worse' is present can be excluded. The individual can be told that he is not 'thick' or lazy and will not be blamed for his 'problem'.

Identification reduces 'learned helplessness' with poor motivation and despondency. The better informed the individual and family are, the less likely they will be to become involved in unorthodox therapies or pathological 'shopping around' (Fox, 1998).

The condition will never get worse, but motor learning may continue to be the area of weakness. Some motor skills may never be learnt, others may be learnt but always be performed badly. Learning may be painful and simple repetition is unlikely to be of benefit. The problems are not

Table 3.4 Assessment tool summary

Physical/ Motor	Visual	Language	Organization/ Attention	Cognitive/ Memory	Independent Living Skills	Social/Emotional Interpersonal
Crawfords Small Parts Dexterity Test	The Beery Buktenica Developmental Test of Visual Motor Integration	Wide Range Achievement Test 3 (WRAT3)	Behavioural Assessment of Dysexecutive Syndrome (BADS)	Wechsler Adult Intelligence Scale – 3rd Edition (WAIS-3)	The Assessment of Motor and Process Skills (AMPS)	Social Use of Language Programme
Grooved Peg Board Test	Test of Visual Perceptual Skills Upper Level (TVPS-UL-R)	Basic Skills Test	Wisconsin Card Sorting Task (WCST-64)	Wide Range Achievement Test 3 (WRAT3)	Canadian Occupational Performance Measure (COPM)	Pragmatic Profile – Adolescents & Adults
Fine Dexterity Test	Motor-Free Visual Perceptual Test (MVPT-3)	Test of Auditory Perceptual Skills (TAPS) (UL)	Brown Attention-Deficit Disorder Scales			Adaptive Behaviour Assessment System (ABAS)
Two Arm Co-ordination Test	Visual Perception Assessment Programme	Test of Adolescent and Adult Language 3rd Ed. (TOAL-3)				Inventory of Interpersonal Problems (IIP-32/IIP-64)
Quick Neurological Screening	Developmental Test of Visual Perception (DTVP–R)	Test of Adolescent/Adult Word Finding (TAWF)				Harters Self-Perception Profile Adolescents and Adults

Table 3.4 continued

Physical/ Motor	Visual	Language	Organization/ Attention	Cognitive/ Memory	Independent Living Skills	Social/Emotional Interpersonal
Aston Postural Assessment	Test of Visual Motor Skills TVMS (UL)	Assessment of Language Related Functional Activities				Becks Depression Inventory – II (BDI – II)
		SCAN-A: A test for Auditory Processing Disorders in Adults				The Awareness of Social Interference Test (TASIT)
						Becks Anxiety Inventory (BAI)

due to lack of intelligence, a history of poor parenting, allergies or active brain disease.

Changed expectations and increased understanding can prove to be helpful in terms of self-esteem as many adults would have passed through their childhood and adolescent years feeling that they were not the same as their peers.

When a diagnosis is given there is a sense of coping with a loss; the order and intensity may vary:

* Numbness – an emptiness
* Anger – frequently displaced to others
* Guilt
* Searching
* Denial
* Depression
* Acceptance

When intervening with an adult with DCD, the professional is likely to need to deal with a range of emotions, attitudes and motivation (also see Chapter 5). Most notable is anxiety; this is a state of apprehension. Anxiety usually concerns the unknown, and relates to the cognitive aspect of emotion. The adult with DCD will need to be kept well informed of his situation in order for him to be relaxed towards any intervention.

> Although it has been very unfortunate that I did not get assessed as a child and so could have had a better chance of managing the condition and exploring my strengths. My worry is that too many with DCD struggle in ignorance, all of their life trying and failing to master basic skills in life and never get the chance (or have the energy left) to discover their often, rare and amazing talents. (Adult with DCD)

Summary

Cermak and Larkin (2001, p. 33) suggest that although a multiple measurement design may be ideal to identify children with DCD before the onset of puberty, it is not clear as yet whether the same design can be applied to those with DCD in adolescence and adulthood. The current diagnostic criteria for developmental disorders in the DSM IV does not take into account the possible change in the manifestation of the disorder with age.

To make an accurate diagnosis of DCD therefore, given that co-morbidity is as high as 60 per cent in young adults and 45 per cent in adults (Portwood, 2000), assessment should include information about the individual's developmental, educational, social and medical history, together with a standardized test of cognitive functioning. The traditional neurological examination is largely unhelpful and any abnormalities seen are not usually associated with DCD and may suggest further investigation or consultation.

Correct identification of DCD in itself constitutes an invaluable intervention. The longstanding anxiety that 'something worse' is present can be excluded. The individual can begin to understand themselves and make sense of their past. A diagnosis can enable individuals to access support in college and work and to become very successful in a chosen career.

CHAPTER 4

Intervention/remediation

The social vs medical model debate – is DCD a disease or a living and learning difficulty?

It has already been discussed in previous chapters that DCD is heterogeneous in nature. Before the matter of assessment is explored it is helpful to consider DCD within 'frames of reference' as this shapes the type of model, e.g. medical or social, that is applied and subsequently the nature of the intervention approaches (see Table 4.1). Various causes of DCD have been investigated and a wide range of approaches has been taken in the identification of the sources of the difficulties experienced (Barnett et al., 1998). Studies to date have centred around brain damage or dysfunction, genetic disposition, impairment in information processing (Cermak and Larkin, 2002). Yet while presenting characteristics of DCD relate to functional difficulties with everyday living (personal, social and emotional) and learning, literature reviews suggest there is little contribution found generally in the assessment or remediation of DCD from social or psychological services.

Words such as 'disorders' and 'disability' tend to be influenced by the medical model, and are also viewed primarily in physical terms, yet it is perfectly possible to have a disability but be highly competent. Conversely it is also possible to have no disability, but yet be quite dysfunctional.

The World Health Organization (WHO) challenges mainstream ideas on how we understand health and disability. ICF (International Classification of Functioning, Disability and Health, 2001) is now an accepted standard to measure health and disability. The ICF shifts the focus to 'life', i.e. how people live with their health conditions and how these can be improved to achieve a productive, fulfilling life. It has implications for medical practice, for law and social policy to improve access and intervention; and for the protection of rights of individuals and groups. Table 4.1 lists a range of common models and frames of reference.

Table 4.1 Models and frames of reference

Frame of reference	Description and functional implications
Medical	Individual is suffering from organic or functional disease, deficit or injury which renders him unable
Environmental	Individual is affected by social and/or environmental barriers, deprivation, or hostile, stressful past or present circumstances
Educational	There is a deficit in learning affecting knowledge, skills or attitudes which consequently affects social or productive performance
Occupational	The individual has an insufficient, or inappropriate, repertoire of necessary occupations and roles, lacks skills or shows occupational imbalance
Developmental	The individual lacks developmental potential and/or has not experienced suitable environmental opportunities to promote development of functional ability
Biomechanical	Strength, range of movement or co-ordination of movement has been affected with consequent limitations of normal function
Neurodevelopmental	The individual shows congenital developmental delay, or delay or regression due to acquired damage to the sensory and nervous system
Cognitive	Problems are due to faulty perception and processing of information, memory, rational thinking, planning, organizing or problem-solving
Analytical	A deficit in, or lack of integration of, the personality resulting from unconscious causes derived from childhood experiences or relationships leading to disturbances of thought, emotion, action or relationships

Source: adapted from Hagedorn (2001).

Table 4.2 World Health Organization dysfunction hierarchy

Term	Interpretation	System
Handicap	Disadvantages for a given individual, resulting from an impairment or a disability, that limits or prevents the fulfilment of a role that is normal (depending on age, sex, and social/cultural factors) for that individual	Social (society, organization, family-group)
Disability	Restriction or lack (resulting from impairment) of ability to perform an activity in the manner or within the range considered normal for a human being	Person
Impairment	Loss or abnormality of psychological, physiological, or anatomical structure or function	Performance

Source: adapted from WHO (1997).

Although there is no 'cure' for DCD there are interventions available that can effectively assist in reducing the 'symptoms'. Just as there is no single test to diagnose DCD, there is no single treatment approach which is appropriate for everyone (Laszlo et al., 1988; Polatajko et al., 1991; Laszlo and Sainsbury, 1993; Revie and Larkin, 1993; Polatajko et al., 1995; Mandich et al., 2001).

It is difficult to categorize and place individuals in discrete intervention/remediation 'boxes'. The multitude of variables of this complex disorder indicates that individuals require a holistic, 'client-centred', multi-faceted and individualized remediation package using a variety of approaches, and ideally within the context of a multi-agency team. Education to colleges, universities, the Department of Work and Pensions and employers about DCD, the difficulties and its management is important for the adult sufferer and their family members.

A multi-dimensional model of intervention

As DCD is a multi-factorial condition it requires a holistic programme that incorporates a spectrum of approaches (Mosey, 1993). They may be used concurrently and/or sequentially.

Table 4.3 A multi-dimensional model of intervention

Approach	Examples	Advantages	Disadvantages
Remedial Emphasizes the facilitation of the improvement of underlying processes	Perceptual motor programmes Movement education Neurodevelopmental treatment on postural motor control	Provides a sense of 'doing something'	Little empirical evidence with regard to effectiveness Difficulty accessing appropriate service providers within locality or nationally
Functional Emphasizes facilitation of the mastery of tasks – skills training	Self-care skills training Social skills training	Deals with immediate issues which affect everyday living and learning skills	Needs skilled professional to teach individual Lack of available resources

Table 4.3 continued

Approach	Examples	Advantages	Disadvantages
Compensatory Emphasizes the minimizing of the effects of the underlying deficits in difficulties in everyday life	Teach coping strategies and study skills Use IT equipment Use specific strategies e.g. colour-coding for perceptual difficulties Set appropriate levels of expectation Allow more time to complete a task	Deals with immediate issues which affect everyday living and learning skills	May make the individual 'feel' or 'look' different from peers or colleagues
Adaptive Emphasizes changing the task or aspects of the environment to minimize the effect of the underlying difficulties	Modification of the environment Use adaptive devices or tools Adapt a specific task	Deals with immediate issues which affect everyday living and learning skills	May make the individual 'feel' or 'look' different from peers or colleagues
Management Emphasizes the minimizing of the distressing or disruptive feelings or behaviour so that the individual can deal with the primary problems	Promote understanding of the problems Consultation with family, employers, tutors Direct intervention toward preventing secondary psycho/social complications	Deals with immediate issues which affect everyday living and learning skills	Need ongoing commitment from those involved with the individual. This may change over time, e.g. change job, line manager leave etc.
Maintenance Emphasis on preserving and supporting the individual's current level of function in a protected environment	Recommend participation in community-based recreational, fitness and social activities Re-assessment and ongoing monitoring of needs	Deal with issues as they arise	Needs commitment from the individual

Principles of intervention

The approach for adults with DCD should:

- *be functional* – focus on activities that are directly relevant to the individual's lifestyle;
- *be goal-based* – goals should be set to maximize potential and prioritized according to the individual's needs;
- *be structured* – may include the need to break down and chain set routines and gradually increase to incorporate longer chains of activity;
- *provide opportunities for errorless learning* – learning is more efficient if a trial and error approach is not permitted but the individual is given cues and prompts which achieve success and are gradually withdrawn;
- *be non-generalized* – opportunities to practise skills in different relevant situations;
- *provide compensation* – offer alternative strategies.

Intervention should:

- be delivered in context, i.e. in a familiar environment at an appropriate time of day needed to facilitate automatic activity;
- facilitate error recognition and compensate appropriately;
- offer visual imagery which may help before an activity is carried out, needed to provide support and reassurance.

Types of intervention for adults with DCD

There is no one best way of remediating DCD. Studies with children have demonstrated that those approaches that incorporated an individualized methodology have had greatest effect. What the research proposes is that professionals keep an open mind to what works best for that individual.

Case-Smith (1998) identifies three themes to intervention:

- Finding the key – looking beyond the outward appearance of the behaviour to find why the problems manifest;
- Sharing information – so that there is a better understanding of behaviours;
- Reframing the behaviour; new awareness produces changes within the living, learning or working environment.

Approaches to intervention for DCD have historically focused on remediation of underlying processing deficits (Laslow and Bairstow, 1985) and facilitating neuro-maturational development (Ayres, 1972), based on the assumption that there is a direct relationship between underlying processes and functional performance. More recent theoretical perspectives have questioned this relationship and there has been a resulting increase in interventions that focus directly on skills acquisition and improved performance (Mandich et al., 2001).

Mandich et al. (2001) suggest that in the absence of strong evidence, professionals need to rely on their judgement to determine the best approach, thereby offering individualized support, using a combination of approaches dependent on need. Although this may seem time-consuming in this day of high caseloads, the lack of sufficient evidence makes it difficult to offer an evidence-based argument for best practice. Therefore the need to develop a systematic, evidence-based approach to intervention is vital, particularly in view of the awareness and identification and increasing understanding regarding the longitudinal picture of DCD.

Fisher (1998) suggests that meaningful occupation is a powerful therapeutic agent and that measuring functional/occupational outcomes is imperative.

Physical intervention

Characteristically, this intervention would be delivered by a chartered physiotherapist who would focus on:

- musculo-skeletal – posture, core stability, flexibility, muscle balance;
- physical stamina, endurance and fitness.

Exercise through the use of leisure activities is also deemed to be helpful, not only for motor skills but also for the other aspects of physical health and well-being. See also Chapter 7.

Occupational therapy (OT)

Occupational therapists are state-registered professionals, usually based with NHS teams or Social Services. The basis of OT is enabling individuals with an illness, injury or disability to be independent in everyday living skills such as home activities, work and community. Therapists take a very practical approach, using a variety of techniques to overcome barriers. Techniques may include teaching individuals new techniques/strategies to approach a task; they may adapt the environment by changing the way a task is done or change the equipment. Some can advise on different aids that can be used as alternatives.

Psychosocial intervention

- *Cognitive behavioural therapy* – This is a form of psychotherapy that emphasizes the important role of thinking in how we feel and what we do. If the individual is experiencing unwanted feelings and behaviours, therapy would help the individual to identify the thinking that is causing the feelings and behaviours and learn how to replace this with more desirable thoughts and reactions.

- *Brief therapy/solution-focused therapy* – This is described as a short-term goal-focused therapeutic approach that helps change by constructing solutions rather than dwelling on problems. Elements of the desired solution are often already present in the individual's life, and become the basis for ongoing change.
- *Behavioural therapy* – This approach is based on the reinforcement of desired behaviours and ignoring the undesired ones. It is an approach that is used within clinical and educational psychology. It is relevant to shaping skill performance.
- *Psychoanalysis* – This is intensive long-term treatment that encourages the individual to explore whatever comes to mind, linking it with events or feelings from earlier experiences. It is not usually available within the NHS.
- *Neuro-linguistic programming (NLP)* – This approach was developed in the 1970s by Bandler and Grinder and developed out of the exploration of the relationship between neurology (brain and its functioning) and linguistics (communication – verbal and non-verbal) and observable patterns (programmes) of behaviour. It has been described as a collection of 'tools' rather than an over-arching theory. NLP consists of a number of 'models' and then 'techniques' based on those models. These include sensory acuity and physiology, the 'meta model', representational systems (based on Erickson's work).
- *Counselling* – A client-centred approach. Counselling sessions are designed to help individuals deal with issues ranging from mental health difficulties, interpersonal conflict and transition, to organization and social skills.
- *Life coaching* – assists the individual to identify the changes they want to make, and assists them in setting their goals. The coach then monitors their progress towards meeting their life changes.

Contemporary approaches

- yoga
- Alexander technique
- Pilates
- aromatherapy
- acupuncture
- herbal remedies

Alternative therapies

- DDAT – This approach aims to remediate symptoms in conditions such as dyslexia, DCD (dyspraxia) and attention deficit disorders. Its approach is based on cerebellar dysfunction that is remediated by a set of prescribed exercises. There are limited empirical studies on the outcome of this approach, and much of the outcome described in the organization's literature is anecdotal.
- INPP – Institute for Neuro-Physiological Psychology. This organization bases its approach on the influence of retained primitive reflexes that are inhibiting the development of movement and learning skills. It offers an assessment and home exercise programme to 'correct specific reflexes'. While some studies have been carried out, there is a lack of strong empirical evidence to support this approach.
- Auditory integration therapy – Based on theories by Dr Berard (a French ENT specialist). Most evidence is based on subjective and unsystematic reports and therefore positive results need to be treated with caution. There is little evidence of long-term benefits. However, there is a positive value in that it encourages individuals to sit quietly and listen, learning to attend. To co-operate to this extent is therefore a major achievement.

Some issues to consider before approaching organizations that provide 'alternative therapies'

It is important to remember there is no such thing as a panacea. Before being tempted by promises of miracles or parting with large amounts of money, individuals and families must be encouraged to seek information on basic issues related to therapy:

About the therapy
- How long has the therapy been used?
- How does the therapy work?
- What types of difficulties do the people who have received this therapy have?
- How many people with DCD or a specific learning difficulty have received this therapy and what were the results?
- What research is available that demonstrates how effective this therapy is for people with DCD and related difficulties?
- How is it decided whether this therapy is appropriate for each individual?
- Will the general practitioner or other professionals be asked for medical/personal history?
- Are there any side-effects and if so what are they?

- How is the outcome of the therapy measured in terms of success?
- Is the therapy unsuitable for certain people and if so for whom and why?
- Will there be follow-up to see if any change has been long-lasting?

About the 'therapist'

- Is the 'therapist' state-registered, and who is the professional body (cite certificates)?
- How long has the 'therapist' been using this therapy or working in this field?
- What training has the 'therapist' undergone and with what institutions, and what qualifications are needed to undergo the training?
- What monitoring is in place to check the quality of the 'therapy' administration?
- What assessments are carried out?
- What evaluation methods will be used to assess the outcome of the treatment?

Drug therapies

At present there is no pharmacological intervention for DCD. Some individuals claim to be helped by taking fish-oil supplements of which an increasing selection is becoming available on the market. Possibly antidepressants or anti-anxiety drugs may be prescribed by the GP.

A pragmatic approach

Task/environmental adaptation

People need to learn through their own efforts; once they learn to do this they can interact with their environment with enthusiasm. Because they need to be encouraged to take the initiative and responsibility for their own learning and experiences, they too should be given opportunities to modify the environment in ways that work for them.

Modifications therefore should not always be seen as external, i.e. designed by someone else for the individual. For the individual to become independent (and to develop self-esteem and confidence) they must encounter the world as it is and learn strategies to solve problems as they come across them. The adult with DCD should have a say in the matter.

The extent and type of adaptation made should be determined on an individual basis. Consider:

- Is this adaptation necessary?
- How will it benefit the individual?

- Is it the least intrusive way of accomplishing the purpose?
- Does it preserve the dignity of the individual?
- What does this say to others – colleagues/students/peers?
- Does this adaptation generalize into the 'natural environment'?
- Have the wishes and desires of the individual been taken into consideration?
- Does this adaptation say to the individual 'you are not able'?

Having analysed the component parts of the activity and its grading prospects it is essential that the professional who is intervening is able to apply the activity/task to the requirements of the individual. In order to do this it may be necessary to change/alter/differentiate the activity or equipment from the usual method of performance to achieve optimum potential.

Adaptations should be, where possible, discussed with both the individual and the family, if appropriate, in order to maintain co-operation. Adaptations should not bewilder nor alarm the individual to the extent they can no longer concentrate on the activity.

Adaptation of activity to compensate for difficulties

- Alter or change the resource/equipment being used
- Eliminate a stage of the activity
- Change the individual's method of doing the activity, e.g. groups to pairs
- Change the teaching method
- Change the environment; change the set-up of the room

Change the individual's skills and ability

- Increase stamina and endurance

General points to consider when choosing an activity/task

Account should be taken of:

- the individual's physical and cognitive level of function;
- the individual's psychological state – motivation, perception and attitudes;
- where the work is to be carried out;
- what time and resources are available.

Problems with this approach

- Workplace/college policy on 'reasonable adjustment' (Disability Discrimination Act 1995) is not clearly articulated (also see Chapter 5).

- Lack of resources
- Timetable/work schedule does not support the staff
- The workplace/college does not support differing learning styles

Environmental considerations (reasonable adjustment)

No matter how enriching an environment is, it is not enriching for the adult with DCD who cannot access it for one reason or another.

At times the pressure to 'fix' the individual, i.e. improve his skills, overshadows the importance of making environmental accommodations. Without appropriate environmental accommodations the individual's motivation and opportunities to become engaged with the environment will be diminished.

Physical structure
The way space is organized (see later chapters for specific strategies).

Examples
- Use pictures to label containers.
- Minimize clutter.
- Ensure routes from one area to another are direct.
- Ensure adequate lighting.

Foster interaction within the environment

Some adults with DCD fail to become engaged in an activity unless there is some guidance.

Examples
- Use modelling, prompting, or physical assistance.
- Remove distracting stimuli.
- Add or enhance visual/verbal cues.

Foster social interaction

Be mindful of the activities presented as some promote/foster particular behaviours. Group size can also influence interaction.

Responsivity

Responsivity provides individuals with predictable and immediate feedback. An environment that allows this helps individuals to acquire a sense of power and security in controlling their environment. It can also be highly motivating and encourages/maintains engagement over time. Adults with DCD who cannot control their environment often develop 'learned helplessness'.

Examples

- Output or performance – adapt how the individual can respond to an instructional task.
- Type of participation – adapt the extent to which the individual is actively involved in the task.
- Expand presentation and delivery of materials – provide more 'hands-on'.
- Provide frequent visual cues to reinforce comprehension.
- Use specific terminology.
- Keep directions/instructions short and simple.
- Speak clearly and face the individual when talking.
- Provide frequent positive feedback.
- Allow time for learning and completion of tasks.

Promoting independence

It is essential to get the balance between fostering independence, i.e. persuading individuals to do things on their own, and ensuring that they are not left out of activities because they lack the required skills.

The following chapters will consider the functional difficulties of the adult with DCD in more detail offering the reader strategies and resources to refer to when working with this group.

Summary

Intervention for DCD has been a great source of debate due to the poorly understood aetiology and competing theories of motor skill development and acquisition (Mandich et al., 2001). There is little in the way of longitudinal studies for adolescents and adults in terms of the likely presenting features; therefore research in terms of intervention is more remote. However, current theories emphasize the importance of contextual factors and that interventions would be more fruitful if they were based on functional activities rather than focusing on the underlying components (Gentile, 1992).

CHAPTER 5
The adult learner

In their study Losse et al. (1991) found that at the age of 16, the children with DCD continued to experience substantial motor difficulties, as well as a variety of educational, social and emotional problems. Academically they were considered to be less successful than their peers despite similar effort. They were also more likely to have lower academic ambitions and a poorer self-concept than their peers. This, it was reported, is likely to affect the type of career choices the individual makes, as he perceives himself to be less able than he may actually be.

Not all educators understand or are responsive to the needs of individuals with learning difficulties such as DCD and related conditions. When teaching methods are not appropriate, people with DCD may become frustrated and experience failure. This may cause them to drop out of educational programmes or make them afraid to enter educational programmes in the first place.

Success at college relies heavily on independent learning skills and demands the ability to deal with many different things at one time. Many will have had a poor experience of learning during their primary and secondary school years, but it is important at this stage for adults with DCD to gain a greater understanding of their strengths and abilities so that they can learn what they need to know, what compensations and accommodations are available to them. Where DCD goes undiagnosed it creates many problems for these individuals. Throughout their time in the education system and on into the workplace, the individual's unique styles of learning may not have been compatible with the traditional teaching styles used in mainstream schools, colleges and companies. This mismatch between the delivery and absorption of information is often the main contributing factor when these individuals do not achieve their potential in the learning environment and ultimately the workplace.

Many with DCD already recognize that others will not understand the nature of their difficulty. It is rarely a lack of ability that causes an adult with DCD to fail at higher or further education, but is more often due to a lack of understanding of the task demands, difficulties with organization and working with their tutors and peers.

Choosing a career

> When I left school at 16, a careers adviser said I was 'non-academic' and should try working in catering. I always tried hard to please so I gave it a go. I did a bakery course, but was just too slow putting the ingredients together. I then moved on to a course on caring for people with learning difficulties and passed with flying colours. At 40 years of age, I am now studying for a diploma in community and youth studies. (Werenowska, 2003, p. 8)

Many individuals have difficulty identifying what type of work or career they would like. The decision can be made a little easier by:

- Gaining a variety of work experiences by doing voluntary work in a number of different types of organizations. For instance, working with animals, on conservation projects, in care homes, with an after-school play scheme, community arts projects, in shops, or going into school, can all help clarify the types of work enjoyed and also help to eliminate some areas.
- Taking a course/courses will help gain experiences and skills that can lead to a job they will enjoy.
- Identifying strengths and what they enjoy doing. This is a good starting point for exploring options.
  - Are they good with people, animals?
  - Are they creative, musical?
  - Are they good with words?
  - Are they good with IT?
  - Are they practical or do they prefer academic work?
- Talking to the careers advisers at school or the disability employment adviser at the local job centre, as they will have information about a wide range of opportunities. They will explore various careers and how their skills and interests match up with them.

Planning for college

When considering going to college or university, there are a number of aspects that need to be considered beforehand.

When to go?

- Is this the right time to go on to higher education or does the individual need a number of stepping-stones to ensure success?
- Is the individual emotionally mature enough to cope with a new course, new town, new university, new friends and new lecturers, or should it be delayed until appropriate skills and support are put in place to increase the chances of success?
- What particular living and learning skills does the individual need to develop in order to promote success, i.e. time management, meal planning and preparation, budgeting, organization, study skills?

Where to go?

- Is a hometown college or one further away more appropriate?
- Is it better for the individual to live independently, or to live at home where there will still be greater support, or is the hall of residence with ready prepared meals a halfway house?
- If the individual wants to go away, is there accessibility to reliable, good road and/or rail services so they can go home easily if they want/need to?
- Does the chosen college have a good Special Needs Support Service or Student Support Service?

Which course?

- Is the chosen course realistic and achievable?
- Can all support structures be in place prior to the start of the course?

What preparation is required?

- Has an application been made for the Disability Students Allowance?
- Are their independent living skills adequate?

Can they:

- plan, shop, prepare a meal and clean up afterwards?
- take care of their personal hygiene, wash clothes, and use an iron? If not able to, what provision is there for help?
- keep their bedroom and study area clean and tidy?
- get up and get to appointments/lectures on time?
- use public transport?
- budget and manage their finances?
- find their way around new places, towns and buildings?
- use appropriate study skills which are adequate for the demands of higher education?

- organize their room, study space, and belongings?
- manage their time and complete assignments in the allotted time?
- use computers to support their studies?

Even with good preparation, college/university life can still be stressful. Some common pitfalls that can lead to stress and frustration are:

- lack of pre-entry planning;
- enrolling in courses that are not suited to the individual or their difficulties;
- taking too many courses at once;
- waiting too long to seek out the services that are needed;
- hesitating to discuss learning needs with the tutors/instructors;
- denying the impact of disability on learning;
- being overwhelmed by the registration process and not asking for help;
- not using time wisely;
- not maintaining a social life;
- poor independent living skills.

Applying for a college/university place

Deciding what to disclose and how much can be difficult. Too much detail could create a negative picture and put off the prospective college. Too little information could result in a college place being given inappropriately, and the individual then needs additional support that has not been planned for. Present difficulties need to be evaluated in order to help identify the appropriate level of support that may be required when undertaking the course.

The individual should arrange for an informal visit to the college/university prior to the interview. This will help them to:

- experience travelling to the place;
- see the surrounding area;
- see/experience the 'working' environment;
- meet people already studying the course and/or studying at the college;
- meet some of the tutors.

The interview

Moving on into college, university or work there will be interviews to attend. Interviews can be stressful situations so it is useful to practise and rehearse interview skills and techniques before the actual day.

Keeping a personal file

Once at college/university the adult with DCD will have to take responsibility for accessing and co-ordinating the support services they need. They will also need to be in control of their personal health and educational information, such as allergies, student support co-ordinator contact details, inoculations and medication etc. A small file that contains all the pertinent information that relates to their health, education and supporting services is valuable.

The file should include information such as:

- any important test scores or information from previous assessments;
- medical documentation which relates to health and any disability;
- a recent IEP (Individual Education Plan) that was developed while in secondary school;
- educational reports;
- letters of recommendation;
- secondary school marks or other official transcripts;
- description of any special testing arrangements or other services that were provided at school, either high school or a post-secondary institution;
- correspondence with funding agencies;
- any information that will help to determine appropriate services that will be needed at college;
- dates of inoculations such as tetanus, hepatitis;
- other services involved.

One adult with DCD reminisces about her time in university:

> I had no problems getting a place at university and was really excited to be starting a degree in modern languages. But as soon as I got on campus everything started to go wrong. It was the practical things that challenged me: close to tears, I would spend up to an hour trying to get the key in the door to my student digs. I could not find my way around the campus and it was a nightmare trying to work out how to use the washing machine or change the duvet on my bed. All of these things were a massive challenge to me so I tried to hide my problems from the other students. I could not even open a bottle of wine or make someone a cup of tea as it would take me so long. After three weeks I suffered a nervous breakdown and had to return home. I felt incredibly bleak and wanted to hide away from the world. I later returned to university and met my husband and got a first class degree.

Figure 5.1 offers a checklist to use with individuals who are considering applying to college or university.

Action point/skill	Comment
Information about HE How to apply What equipment, resources and support systems are available What are the learning, teaching and assessment styles The level and amount of work required Expectations of studying What are the benefits of declaring a disability or special educational need Can the prospective student apply for DSA?	
Skills and abilities that may be required Study skills, note-taking, research skills Independent learning skills Independent living skills Self-advocacy, self-motivation, assertiveness, negotiation skills Self-awareness – including judging own potential and performance Realistic goal setting Demonstrate an ability to meet the demands of the course Flexibility, coping skills, time management Budgeting Stress management Using communication and information technology Ability and confidence to ask appropriate questions	
Preparation Advice and help to fill in forms Help with investigation of courses Visits to institution Accurate impartial assessment of need Detailed induction Help completing DSA application and managing allowance Support in place at the start of the course Opportunity to practise with support workers and/or equipment Time to learn and use equipment and discover layout of buildings Links with role models Sympathetic and trained staff	

Figure 5.1 Checklist for prospective students.

The law and education relating to students with DCD

The Disability Discrimination Act 1995 (DDA) was extended to education from September 2002 following amendments introduced by the Special Educational Needs and Disability Act 2001. The legislation aimed to ensure that disabled people, and that includes DCD and related conditions such as dyslexia, have equal opportunities to benefit from, and contribute to, the learning and services available in higher education institutions.

A brief outline of institutions' responsibilities

The Act makes it unlawful to discriminate against disabled applicants, potential applicants or students. The Act uses a wide definition of disabled person. It can include people with:

- physical or mobility impairments
- visual impairments
- hearing impairments
- dyslexia
- medical conditions, and
- mental health difficulties.

Discrimination against disabled applicants or students can take place in either of two ways. By:

- treating them 'less favourably' than other people, or
- failing to make a 'reasonable adjustment' when they are placed at a 'substantial disadvantage' compared to other people for a reason relating to their disability.

The Act applies to all the activities and facilities institutions providing wholly or mainly for students, including, for example:

- all aspects of teaching and learning, including lectures, lab work, practical work, field trips, work placements etc.;
- e-learning, distance learning;
- examinations and assessments;
- learning resources, including libraries, computer facilities etc.;
- aspects of the physical environment such as buildings, landscaping and equipment;
- welfare, counselling and other support services;
- catering, residential and leisure facilities;
- careers services.

A reasonable adjustment might be any action that helps to alleviate a substantial disadvantage. It might involve:

- changing standard institutional procedures;
- adapting the curriculum, electronic or other materials, or modifying the delivery of teaching;
- providing additional services, such as a sign language interpreter or materials in Braille;
- training staff to work with disabled people and to provide appropriate adjustments;
- altering the physical environment.

See also Chapter 4.

Institutions are only expected to do what is 'reasonable'. What is reasonable will depend on all the individual circumstances of the case, including the importance of the service, the financial or other resources of the institution and the practicality of the adjustment. Other issues, such as the need to maintain academic standards, health and safety and the relevant interests of other people including other students are also important.

Knowledge of students' disabilities and confidentiality

Institutions are expected to take reasonable steps to find out about a student's disability. Once a student has disclosed a disability, even if only to one staff member, or once an institution might reasonably be expected to know about a student's disability (for example, if it is visible), the institution has a responsibility not to discriminate. Students do, of course, have a right to confidentiality, both through the Data Protection Act 1998, and separately within the Disability Discrimination Act.

Issues to cover

Different staff groups will need to cover different aspects of the DDA or of good practice. Wherever possible, it is useful to tailor training to individual needs.

- Senior managers and heads of departments need to have a thorough understanding of their legal responsibilities. Other staff may need only a brief outline of the law.
- Staff with management responsibility need to know how to make anticipatory adjustments in their departments.
- All staff who come into direct contact with disabled students and applicants need to know how to respond to a student who discloses a disability.
- All staff who come into direct contact with disabled students need to know how they can make appropriate adjustments for disabled people.
- All members of staff need to know who, within the institution, can offer further advice and information. It may be helpful if one staff member in each department can receive more comprehensive training so that they can act as an initial point of contact.
- All staff need to know that they personally have a responsibility towards disabled students.
- Specific staff may need training 'top-up' sessions in, for example, how to support a student having an epileptic seizure, or how to communicate with a hard-of-hearing person.

Other issues to consider

Many people have an emotional response to disability. They may have entrenched attitudes based on prejudice or previous negative (or positive) experiences. For this reason, it may be harder to change attitudes and behaviours relating to disability than other issues.

The Human Rights Act 1998 includes the 'right to education' and sits alongside the Disability Discrimination Act inasmuch as the Act states that there is a 'prohibition of discrimination'.

Presenting difficulties for students with DCD and suggestions for reasonable adjustment

The following table lists potential areas of difficulty which may be experienced by students with DCD. The table also offers some suggestions to enable the student to learn and study more effectively.

Table 5.1 Presenting features and adjustment

Area of difficulty	Functional difficulties	Adjustment
Memory (Immediate/ short-term/long-term memory) Reading from text Listening	Confusion or lose track of what has been said or have difficulty following instructions Difficulty with simultaneous note-taking and listening in lectures Weak attention and concentration Forget what has been read immediately after reading it Take a long time to extract and retain information when reading material Lose track of what is being said while listening to it	Provide opportunities and support to develop study skills techniques such as: • Creating brain frames – Mind Maps or Spider Diagrams • Using flash cards – (Index/ Postcards) • Highlighting and underlining • Using mnemonics Provide handouts or copy OHP slides from lectures Allow individual time to process and answer question Provide Dictaphones to record lectures Assess for appropriate computer hardware and software Provide a reader

Table 5.1 continued

Area of difficulty	Functional difficulties	Adjustment
Organization	Losing papers, possessions, incomplete assignments	Use of small aids such as stopwatches and alarms
	Difficulties with tasks under time pressure	Use an electronic organizer with stylus operation such as a 'Palm Pilot', 'Compaq'
	Difficulties undertaking a series of tasks at once – problem-solving	Use a notice board/pin board to pin up reminders and a 'To do' job list
	Essay-writing – difficulty organizing thoughts into a clear and coherent piece of writing	Provide a mentor to help prioritize what needs to be done that day/week and what can wait
	Difficulty with peer presentations	Provide Dictaphone, talking pen or mini-microphone to record things that are easily forgotten. Use a buddy or classroom assistant to help plan work out
	Difficulty restarting a task once interrupted	
	Failure to meet deadlines	Allow greater time to complete tasks, understand task components, grade activities, model what is required, give feedback
		Creation of opportunities to learn and develop study skills – use of flow charts and/or bullet points to summarize information and key points
		Provide 'templates'
Communication Talking, listening, social and communication skills	Talking too much, repeating information, and 'going off at a tangent'.	Give clear instructions
		Give information in a written format
	Long pauses in mid-sentence and not being able to find the right words or way of expressing thoughts	Use demonstration and gestural cues to support verbal instructions
		Re-frame instructions
		Use visual schemas to support the expression of thoughts and ideas
	Not appropriately initiating and ending conversations	
	Interrupting people or taking over their speech	

Table 5.1 continued

Area of difficulty	Functional difficulties	Adjustment
Communication	Failure to demonstrate listening has taken place by giving replies which are not entirely relevant to what the other person has said	
	Not picking up non-verbal communication	
	Not understanding jokes, idiom, sarcasm or metaphor	
Academic Reading, writing, spelling, numbers	Reading can be slower than average and word decoding difficulties may lead to poor comprehension of what has been read	Teach study skills Provide a reader Provide a scribe Assess for appropriate ICT and small aids
	Producing fluent and concise notes/projects is often problematic. Often the well-organized thoughts of the person with DCD become disorganized as they write them down.	

Special arrangements

It is quite likely that a student with DCD is eligible for special arrangements for examinations.

Special arrangements depend on the degree of functional difficulty and
the examining board. These could be:

- additional reading time;
- additional working time;
- enlarged print on the exam paper;
- coloured exam paper;
- use of computers;
- a reader;
- a scribe;
- provision of a separate room in which to take the exam.

Disability Students Allowance (DSA)

This grant can help with costs incurred in attending a course as a direct result of the disability. It is not related to income and does not have to be repaid. There are four main types of financial help:

- specialist equipment allowance
- non-medical helper allowance
- general disabled student allowance
- extra travel cost allowance

A useful guide to accessing DSA is *Bridging the Gap: a Guide to the Disabled Students Allowance* (DfES, 2003).

Technology and DCD

The use of technology for students with DCD within a learning environment can be extremely helpful. However, any equipment needs to fit into the requirements of the course and, most importantly, be relevant to the needs of the individual with DCD. Table 5.2 compares and contrasts the advantages and disadvantages of using technology for students with DCD.

Table 5.2 Technology and DCD: advantages and disadvantages

Advantages	Disadvantages
Motivator for a previously failed task	Poor organizational difficulties may impact on responsibility for looking after equipment
Provides opportunities for over-learning	Sequencing and problem-solving skills for accessing programmes may impact on using ICT to full potential
Immediate response	
Can dictate pace	Cost
Adaptable for the learner	Changing pace of technology
Wide range of programmes available	Training
Portable systems available	May need to be compatible with the institution's resources/technical support
Speed	
Presentation	Insurance
Organizing tool	

In order for the adult with DCD to get the most out of their computer they should be able to:

- store and retrieve documents in files in a systematic way;
- set up templates;
- use shortcuts on the desktop to access files;
- use search modes;
- use auto-correct;

- use abbreviation facility;
- use word prediction facility;
- use homophones (words that sound similar, but are spelt differently, e.g. bare, bear) facility;
- use the thesaurus and spell-checker facility;
- set up useful phrases and spellings.

The table below lists some adaptations and suggestions to enable easier computer access for students with DCD.

Table 5.3 Examples of computer solutions for students with DCD

Keyboards	Mouse	Screen	Software
Sticky keys	Ergonomic	Adjust screen resolution	Text-to-speech
Key repeat rate	mouse	Increase size and type of	Speech-to-text
Key Guards	Tracker balls	font	Magnifiers
Different size	Pen devices	Word predication	Study and
keyboards	Increase size	Change/customize	learning
Keyboard layout	and speed	Windows colour scheme	tools
'qwerty'/alphabetical	of mouse	Magnifier (Window98ME)	Concept
Ergonomic keyboards	pointer	Configure Web-browser	organizers
Keyboard position		Text cursor	Typing tutors
Laptop			
Palmtop			

Summary

Studies in which the development of academic competence in individuals with DCD has been examined are relatively rare (Cermak and Larkin, 2002). However, what is known from the limited studies is that despite average IQ, academic progress is at risk. For many individuals, educational problems may be focal or causal in a difficult journey to adulthood (Grove and Giraud-Saunders, 2003).

For those entering further or higher education with a diagnosis, they can often obtain practical and financial support from the outset. In some incidences, entering college or university is the first time that difficulties or issues with learning have been acknowledged or identified. In this case, the impact on the individual can have the effect of being able to make sense of a turbulent educational past. The Special Needs and Disability Act (DfES, 2001) appears to have opened doors to further education opportunities (Clark, 2003). This, together with a growing awareness of specific learning difficulties such as DCD insofar as they are not solely childhood disorders, has meant that the needs of those individuals who learn differently can be accommodated and supported, leading to successful achievements in their studies.

CHAPTER 6

The adult at work

DCD and barriers to achievement

Employment provides an economic means, gives social status and promotes social inclusion (Davies and Rinaldi, 2004). While many adults with DCD attach a high priority to gaining and retaining employment, they can also face many barriers.

Knuckey and Gubbay (1983) found that adolescents with extreme motor problems had the least skilled jobs. This was further supported by Losse et al. (1991), who reported that by the age of 16, adolescents diagnosed with DCD at 6 years of age not only had lower school achievement, but as a consequence, some of them found it hard to gain employment (Cantell, 1998).

Employment is often thought of as a means to an end, with the main function that of providing a living. However there are many other side benefits. It necessitates a time structure on the waking day, and implies shared regular contacts with others outside of the 'family'. It also defines 'status' and identity (Jahoda, 1979).

Evidence also suggests that unemployment has negative health consequences. In his work, Warr (1984) provided evidence that the adverse effects of unemployment resulted in: increased apathy, indecision, inability to structure daytime and leisure activities, loss of social contact and loss of self-esteem. Furthermore, Lewis and Slogett (1998) found in their research that there was a relationship between unemployment and an increased risk of suicide.

DCD is not an intellectual difficulty, nor does it imply that there are only difficulties with co-ordination and organizational skills. More significantly in adulthood, its secondary effect of low self-esteem has damaging consequences for social and psychological development. The role of purposeful employment therefore, whether that be voluntary or paid employment, is important in the life of an adult with DCD.

DCD is only a relatively recently acknowledged disability within medical circles, let alone in the areas of further/higher education and employment. As a result adults with DCD have to struggle to cope within the workplace because not only have employers not been able to understand the effects of the condition, but the individuals themselves may not be aware of all the manifestations of DCD. As a consequence, holding down a job or progressing along a career pathway has been beset by barriers.

Lament of a Dyspraxic

I'm uncompromisingly uncoordinated
It makes me angry and frustrated.
You may smile and say, 'well, well'.
But I cannot write and I cannot spell.
I cannot do a lot of things
You should feel the sense of failure it brings.
When I was small, – a child at school
They called me stupid, a dunce, a fool!
I was bad at sports, I couldn't spell my name,
They thought I was playing some kind of 'game'!
I couldn't tell the time, nor tie a shoelace.
The embarrassment of failing made me go red in the face.
Though I was intelligent, and sometimes bright,
I failed to distinguish left from right!
Memorizing the alphabetical sequence, I was completely unable,
I also failed to learn and recite any mathematical table!
I was always singled out as a stupid kid
By this failure to learn and the things I did.
Confused, as on to what I could 'lay the blame'
Of course this cursed affliction that filled me with shame.
Destroying my confidence and spoiling my life
Consigning me to the scrap heap, and thus financial strife.
Not only my confidence did it rob,
But has made me unfit to do a proper job!
But now that I'm older, informed and wise
This disability is partially caused by my brain and my eyes.
Learning difficulties, with poor co-ordination,
Have caused me pain, anguish and years of frustration.
So instead of reaching for pills or the rope
I must help myself and learn to cope.
But I need some employer to help me and give me a chance
To improve my life and happiness advance

With permission: Shirley Hastings (Werenowska, 2003, p. 49).

To tell or not to tell

DCD is often referred to as a 'hidden disability' with difficulties being less obvious and less well understood. Many individuals with DCD and related conditions struggle with the issue of 'disclosure', i.e. whether to tell the employer or not. Also, as already suggested, many realize they have difficulties but do not understand why.

Should an individual wish to disclose their condition to their employer, the timing and delivery can be quite crucial. The following should be considered:

* Who should be told
* When should it be said
* Why should it be said
* How should it be said
* What should be said

The following table compares reasons to disclose or not to disclose information to employers.

Table 6.1 Disclosure to employers

Reasons to disclose	Reasons not to disclose
If false information is given on job application, the employee may face dismissal and is later identified	DCD may not affect the individual's ability to do the job
Many employers have equal opportunity policies and are committed to employing those with disabilities	If job competition is fierce disclosure may place the individual with DCD at a disadvantage
The individual may be less nervous at interview	Employer may focus on DCD as a disability instead of on strengths
Reasonable adjustment can be made	The employer may doubt the ability of the individual to perform the role thereby creating a poor work environment
Reduce any later embarrassment	The individual may have difficulty gaining promotion
Understanding from colleagues	
By law the individual with DCD cannot be dismissed because of the condition	
Less stress as the individual does not have to 'hide' the 'disability'	

The law and services to support adults with DCD in employment

The Disability Discrimination Act 1995 (DDA) now offers some protection and resources for the employee with DCD. The DDA defines a person with a disability as having:

A physical or mental impairment which has a severe long-term adverse effect on a person's ability to carry out normal day-to-day activities.

The Employment Service can offer a wide range of schemes designed to help individuals with employability and job retention.

- The Disability Services Team provides specialist help and advice for people with disabilities and their employers.
- Work psychologists. These professionals work within the Disability Services Division and provide specialist assessment, counselling and training for people with disabilities.
- Access to Work and Disability Employment Advisors (DEAs). These professionals are based in job centres and are engaged to help and advise individuals who are encountering barriers to employment because of their disabilities. They work with the occupational psychologists and can help with:
  - assessment of abilities and the type of job which may suit the individual. A plan of action is drawn up regarding obtaining employment or to attend relevant training courses.
  - contact – able to put individuals in touch with prospective employers.
  - Access to Work – this is a programme to make the most of opportunities in the workplace by providing a range of assistance to overcome obstacles caused by the disability, e.g. support worker, equipment, alteration to the work environment.

The Employment Service offers a number of programmes such as New Deal, which is designed to help unemployed people generally, but has specific provision for people with disabilities.

Individuals with DCD should look out for employers who use the disability symbol on job advertisements, application forms and recruitment literature. It shows that a company is positive about employing disabled people.

Reasonable adjustment

Under the DDA, employers have certain duties to make 'reasonable adjustment' to ensure that adults with DCD are not placed at a substantial disadvantage by their employment arrangements or by any physical feature of the workplace.

Reasonable adjustments are accommodations, methods, techniques, strategies and workplace adaptations that enable the individual to perform their job.

Examples of adjustment employers should consider:

- making adjustments to the building;
- allocating some of the employee's work to someone else;
- transferring the employee to another post or other place of work;
- being flexible about hours – allowing the employee to be away from the job for interventions, e.g. assessment/treatment;
- providing training;
- using modified equipment;
- making instructions and manuals more accessible;
- using a reader or interpreter.

Managers have a key role in enabling employees with DCD to work at a level commensurate with their ability. They need to be clear as to what they are expecting from the individual and what can be achieved through the right adjustments. They need to remember that in general adults with DCD:

- process information differently;
- can lack confidence and be reluctant to ask questions;
- often perform less well in written tasks than is expected;
- can be defensive in new training situations because of their past experience;
- always need positive feedback;
- have skills and abilities that they do not recognize for themselves.

One adult with DCD reported . . .

> In 9 years I was redeployed four times. It was always the same – 'you're nice but unsuitable'.

By understanding their difficulties and potential problems employers can plan ahead in order to match the individual's skills to the job/task and to provide the support and encouragement that the employee with DCD needs. This will help to minimize potential problems and enable the individual to function more effectively and efficiently in their work. An understanding boss will be flexible in their approach and will be able to identify alternative ways of working which are suitable to the individual's situation.

Table 6.2 outlines the potential difficulties that employees with DCD can experience in their work.

Table 6.2 Difficulties within the workplace

Difficulties with memory

Area of difficulty	Functional implications
Names, labels, numbers	Take longer than average (or failing completely) to learn the names of colleagues. This often results in the employee with DCD avoiding using names and/or using wrong names. Inability to remember/confusing dates and times, e.g. appointments and meetings. Forget telephone numbers to the extent that they cannot repeat the number immediately after hearing it. Forget codes and passwords for doors, photocopiers, computer systems.
Sequences	Unable to give accurate directions or follow directions given by others. Unable to retain instructions given verbally, for example a list of tasks given by a supervisor. Unable to learn from written instructions the sequence of behaviours required for standard procedures.
Reading text	Forget what has been read immediately after reading it. Take a long time to extract and retain information when reading material.
Listening	Forget what has been said, or most of it, almost immediately after hearing it. Lose track of what is being said while listening to it.
Taking messages	Forget important parts of the message. Confuse or reverse information provided in messages.
Organization	Lose personal belongings such as keys, pens, wallet etc. Lose materials especially if the employee with DCD is working in several different places. Difficulty budgeting and managing their money.

Difficulties with communication

Area of difficulty	Functional implications
Talking	Talk too much, repeating information, and 'going off at a tangent'. Long pauses in mid-sentence and not being able to find the right word. Poor pronunciation, particularly of long words. Not appropriately initiating and ending conversations.
Listening	Interrupt people or taking over their speech. Fail to demonstrate listening has taken place by giving replies that are not entirely relevant to what the other person has said.

Table 6.2 continued

Difficulties with communication

Area of difficulty	Functional implications
Social and communication skills	Not following unwritten social rules and acceptable behaviour such as social distance. Not picking up non-verbal communication. Not understanding jokes, idiom, sarcasm and metaphor. Difficulty clearly expressing ideas and thoughts.
Messages	Give confusing or garbled verbal messages.
Reading, writing and spelling	Reading can be slower than average and word decoding difficulties may lead to poor comprehension of what has been read. Producing fluent and concise material is often problematic. Often the well-organized thoughts of the person with DCD become disorganized as they write them down. Making notes and/or taking minutes of meetings is difficult due to having to multi-task – listen, pick out key points, while recording information at the same time.

Difficulties with organization and self-management

Area of difficulty	Functional implications
Attention	Easily distracted by noise, objects and people.
Completing unfinished tasks	Have difficulty restarting a task once interrupted. Often adults with DCD cannot recall where they were up to and may have to go back to the beginning or may start at the wrong place that results in omissions and errors.
Time management	Often fail to leave enough time to complete a task or a journey, or do not realize how long a job has taken them to do. Failure to meet deadlines is common. Frequently being late for work, completing tasks in time, and/or keeping to specified break times.
Paperwork	General disorganization, poor filing, sorting and untidiness are common. Not getting paperwork done is common. Adults with DCD often put off or avoid paperwork and report writing whenever possible.

Table 6.2 continued

Difficulties with co-ordination

Area of difficulty	Functional implications
Balance and co-ordination	Clumsy gait and movement. Poor quality and control of movement. Overflow and exaggerated accessory movements may be visible. Difficulty riding a bike and driving a car that may affect independent travel to the workplace.
Fine motor control	Poor manual dexterity, leading to difficulties with keyboard skills, operating machinery and equipment, unscrewing things, opening doors and locks and fiddly or intricate tasks. Difficulty with handwriting; the employee with DCD may have a poor pen grip, may not finish off words, nor keep on the line, and/or press too hard. Difficulty fastening buttons and zips, putting on make-up and combing own hair can lead to poor personal appearance. Appear clumsy and frequently drop things and may unintentionally break equipment.
Poor posture and reduced stamina	Weak muscle tone and muscle strength especially around the pelvis and shoulders and therefore at risk of neck and back problems.
Poor body awareness	Tendency to fall, trip over and bump into things and people.
Multi-tasking	Difficulty doing more than one task at a time such as listening, watching and doing.

Success at work depends on several factors; these include:

- knowing one's own abilities and skills;
- knowing what the demands of the job are;
- feeling comfortable within the environment;
- having the chance to use one's skills and knowing that they are valued;
- support of colleagues to help overcome and/or alleviate problems;
- the ability to reflect on and evaluate one's performance.

A work performance rating scale could be used by managers and supervisors to help identify the employee's strengths and the areas where they experience difficulty. Once these have been highlighted it is important for the manager to consider how these difficulties may impact on the individual's performance at work. Carrying out a job analysis of the individual's specific roles and duties within the organization can assist in this process. A task analysis is a technique through which demands of specific jobs are identified and analysed and is considered by some to be essential to effective performance at work (McLoughlin et al., 2002).

Employee's Name ....Area of Work...

Line Manager...   Date.............................

Read both sets of statements and circle the number that most accurately describes the employee:

Task Competence		
Does complicated jobs well	5 4 3 2 1	Prefers to do simple tasks
Grasps instructions quickly	5 4 3 2 1	Can't grasp instructions
Pace of work is satisfactory	5 4 3 2 1	Pace of work is not satisfactory
Needs little supervision of work	5 4 3 2 1	Needs constant supervision
Always uses good judgement	5 4 3 2 1	Hardly ever uses good judgement
Achieves an excellent standard of work	5 4 3 2 1	Achieves a poor standard of work
Manual dexterity is good	5 4 3 2 1	Manual dexterity is poor
Uses tools/equipment well	5 4 3 2 1	Can't use tools/equipment
Responses to Authority and Supervision		
Welcomes supervision	5 4 3 2 1	Dislikes supervision
Willing to change jobs	5 4 3 2 1	Not willing to change jobs
Has a sensible attitude to authority	5 4 3 2 1	Has a poor attitude to authority
Accepts criticism/correction of work	5 4 3 2 1	Can't accept criticism/correction
Work Motivation and Enthusiasm		
Works to times set	5 4 3 2 1	Has problems working to times set
Eager to work	5 4 3 2 1	Avoids work
Looks for more work	5 4 3 2 1	Waits to be given work
A good time-keeper	5 4 3 2 1	A poor time-keeper
Has a good record of attendance	5 4 3 2 1	Has a poor record of attendance
I would be willing to employ him/her	5 4 3 2 1	I would prefer not to employ him/her
Always finishes the work	5 4 3 2 1	Leaves the work unfinished
Confidence and Initiative		
Takes a prominent part in things	5 4 3 2 1	Hangs back letting others take lead
Is happy to help others	5 4 3 2 1	Is unable/unwilling to help others
Is markedly over-confident (5 = realistic)	2 3 5 3 2	Is markedly under-confident
Accepts responsibilities very readily	5 4 3 2 1	Can't readily accept responsibility
Relationships with Others		
Gets on well with others	5 4 3 2 1	Does not get on well with others
Communicates spontaneously	5 4 3 2 1	Communication is poor
Likes working in a team	5 4 3 2 1	Prefers to work alone
Personal Organizational Skills		
Needs no prompting to start work	5 4 3 2 1	Needs prompting to start work
Organizes his/her work effectively	5 4 3 2 1	Doesn't organize work effectively
Organizes work space effectively	5 4 3 2 1	Doesn't organize work space effectively
Organizes self effectively	5 4 3 2 1	Doesn't organize self effectively
Has appropriate personal grooming	5 4 3 2 1	Inappropriate personal grooming
Has appropriate appearance at work	5 4 3 2 1	Inappropriate appearance at work
Asks for help when needed	5 4 3 2 1	Doesn't ask for help when needed

Source: Anon.

Figure 6.1 An example of a work performance rating scale.

The results of the job analysis need to be considered alongside the skills, abilities and difficulties of the individual with DCD in order that they may be given the opportunity to work at a level that matches their ability.

Having completed the task analysis and an employee's performance rating scale, it is important to identify and assess areas of potential risk for the individual. For example some employees with DCD continue to have poor co-ordination and manual dexterity and will be at risk of injury in some types of employment where the use of machinery and/or sharp equipment is a significant part of the duties.

A risk assessment is nothing more than a careful examination of that which could cause harm to people, in this instance in the workplace. Employers have a legal responsibility to assess the risks in their workplace and to consider whether adequate precautions have been taken or whether more needs to be done to prevent harm. The general aim is to make sure, as far as possible, that no one gets hurt or becomes ill.

Table 6.3 gives the five steps of risk assessment; this is a useful framework to use when carrying out risk assessments for an employee with DCD.

Table 6.3 Steps to risk assessment

STEP 1	Look for the hazards / difficulties
STEP 2	Decide who might be harmed and how
STEP 3	Evaluate the risks and decide whether the existing precautions are adequate or whether more should be done
STEP 4	Record your findings
STEP 5	Review your assessment and revise it if necessary

People with DCD respond well to routines, structures and having instructions stated clearly and concisely. Table 6.4 lists some practical suggestions as to how employers and line managers can help the individual with DCD to reach their potential within their workplace. These suggestions are valid regardless of whether the individual is in paid employment or is 'working' in a voluntary capacity.

Table 6.4 Practical suggestions on how employers can help the individual with DCD to reach their potential within their workplace

Workplace setting	Job requirements	Factors to consider/ potential areas of difficulty	Adjustment
Office	Filing	Fine motor skills – grips, grasps	Use a pin board to hold important information.
	Organization of self	Gross motor skills – moving and handling	Use 'To do' lists
	Organization of workload	Safety awareness	Colour-coded/labelled files and folders
	Organization of work space	Posture - sitting, work station ergonomics	Use desk and drawer tidies
	Time management	Problem-solving	Use see-through containers or clear files to store documents
	Using telephone	Sequencing	Use transparent pencil cases/purses so the contents can be easily seen
	Multi-tasking – auditory/motor skills	Priority setting, time management	Use computer directories and facilities to support job requirements
	Using office equipment – fax, photocopier	Completing tasks	Create a 'message pad' template with key words/ prompts to make taking telephone messages easier
	Using ICT	Literacy, numeracy	Draw up 'templates' of report formats/letters
	Handwriting	Appearance	Use different coloured floppy disks for different/specific projects
	Record keeping, statistics	Social skills	Use a dictaphone, talking pen or mini-microphone to record things that are easily forgotten
	Relationships – with peers, managers, subordinates	Attention, concentration	Devise step-by-step instructions for different operating procedures
	Following instructions	Motivation	Consider providing software that converts speech into text and vice versa
	Meeting targets and deadlines	Self-esteem, confidence	Allow the employee to use earplugs or a headset to cut out noise
	Remembering instructions and procedures	Managing stress	Use answerphones or voice-mail to control phone calls
		Punctuality	Use a 'page a day' diary
		Absence record	Customize computer – fonts/background

Table 6.4 continued

Workplace setting	Job requirements	Factors to consider/ potential areas of difficulty	Adjustment
Retail	Filling shelves Stacking Stocktaking Customer services Checkout operation Handling money Administration and form-filling Following instructions – managers/ supervisor Following procedures Initiating Multi-tasking Relationships with colleagues	Fine motor skills – grips, grasps Moving and handling Safety awareness Posture Fitness, stamina – standing for long periods Problem-solving Sequencing Priority setting, time management Completing tasks Literacy, numeracy, comprehension Appearance Social skills Attention, concentration Motivation Self-esteem, confidence Managing stress Punctuality Absence record	Provide a dictaphone, talking pen or mini-microphone to record things that are easily forgotten Keep copies of step-by-step instructions for different operating procedures – make them small enough to fit in a pocket i.e. laminated credit card size Use 'To do' lists and tick off items when they have been completed Clearly label the stockroom – label shelves, drawers, cupboards, using colour codes, pictures or large print. Create a map of the stockroom layout / shop layout Create a photograph board of all the employees Create a flow chart for specific duties Keep regular routines so that they become a habit Provide regular supervision Colour-code forms and paperwork Encourage the employee to ask for help and not to hide mistakes Provide good seating if sitting for long periods
Manual labour	Using equipment and tools – drills, hammers Operating large machinery Assembling – goods	Health and safety Risk assessment Problem-solving Social skills Comprehension Attention, concentration	Move to other duties – i.e. requiring less speed, less dexterity, less stamina Consider alternative working positions Ensure correct health and safety procedures

Table 6.4 continued

Workplace setting	Job requirements	Factors to consider/ potential areas of difficulty	Adjustment
Manual labour (contd)	Following verbal instructions – managers/ supervisor Team working Multi-tasking Meeting targets and deadlines Assessing risks	Motivation Self-esteem, confidence Managing stress Punctuality Absence record Gross motor skills, stamina	Keep copies of step-by-step instructions for different operating procedures – make them small enough to fit in a pocket i.e. laminated credit card size Adaptation – putting in additions to existing environment – pulleys, handles, painting with contrasting colours, bell instead of visual cue, lighting Alter level of working height
Factory	Using equipment and tools Sustain repetitive actions at speed Assembling – goods Following verbal instructions Meeting individual targets	Fitness, stamina – standing for long periods Sequencing Literacy, numeracy, comprehension Social skills Attention, concentration	Move to other duties – i.e. requiring less speed, sitting instead of standing Reduce stress Adaptation – putting in additions to existing environment – pulleys, handles, painting with contrasting colours, bell instead of visual cue, lighting Alter level of working height

(Refer to Chapter 5 for the use of ICT and the adult with DCD.)

Other work opportunities

On occasions it is too daunting or difficult for individuals with DCD to cope in the workplace. The following may be alternatives for consideration:

- Voluntary work – this can build the bridge into paid employment and provide references, proving skills and abilities
- Working from home
- Self-employment
- Supported employment
- Job introduction schemes

Summary

Employment plays a key role in people's lives; it offers time structure to the waking day and implies shared regular contacts with others outside of the 'family'. It also defines 'status' and identity. Unemployment can result in increased apathy, indecision, inability to structure daytime and leisure activities, loss of social contact and loss of self-esteem. Individuals with DCD have been found to have lower school achievement, and as a consequence, some of them find it hard to gain employment.

It is important to remember that many individuals with DCD are not unintelligent but have an IQ that is average or above, and have many valuable skills and abilities that are important to the work of any organization. In order to help them work to their potential it is important to increase their self-confidence and belief in their own abilities. In this way the adult with DCD can be a valued and essential member of a team.

The employer/line manager should therefore:

- give praise and show appreciation whenever relevant;
- show confidence in their abilities;
- recognize and acknowledge their talents and their strengths;
- avoid making harsh criticisms or careless remarks that could undermine their confidence;
- remember what DCD is and what it is not. Individuals with DCD are not lazy or stupid;
- many people with DCD find written and organizational work much harder than their peers and colleagues; generally they put a great deal more energy and concentration into written and organizational work than other people;
- let the employee know that their difficulties are understood and that the organization wants to support and help them;

- encourage the employee to be open about their difficulties rather than hide them;
- remember that late reports or absenteeism may result from fear and from feeling overwhelmed by tasks;
- recognize that reluctance to apply for promotion and/or training courses is often linked to low confidence in their abilities;
- make reasonable adjustments.

CHAPTER 7

The adult at play

Social and emotional implications of DCD

Numerous studies have examined the social, emotional and behavioural problems associated with motor difficulties, leading to a growing body of evidence that the lack of movement skills may have damaging consequences for social and psychological development. Research also suggests that these individuals are at risk of withdrawing from physical activities resulting in a further impairment of motor skills and a negative impact on physical fitness, health and well-being.

Given that motor competence is positively related to social acceptance (Rose et al., 1997), it is not surprising that those with DCD occupy marginal positions within their peer groups and have few 'playmates' (Clifford, 1985; Kalverboer et al., 1990; Schoemaker and Kalverboer, 1994). When participation in group activities does occur, those who lack the motor competencies are frequently the target of criticism and ridicule. As a result individuals with DCD withdraw. Continued avoidance of participation in activities leads to feelings of unhappiness, exclusion and isolation.

A sense of guilt and shame

As already discussed in previous chapters, individuals growing up with DCD often feel a sense of shame. For some, it is a great relief to receive the diagnosis while for others the label only serves to further stigmatize them.

Sadly, these feelings of shame often cause the individual to hide their difficulties. Rather than risk being labelled as stupid or accused of being lazy, some adults deny their learning disability as a defence mechanism. Internalized negative labels of stupidity and incompetence usually result in a poor self-concept and lack of confidence (Gerber et al., 1992).

Fear

Fear is another emotional difficulty for adults with DCD. This emotion is often masked by anger or anxiety.

Feelings of fear may be related to one or more of the following issues:

* fear of being found out;
* fear of failure;
* fear of judgment or criticism, ridicule;
* fear of rejection.

Being found out

Many adults with DCD live with fear of being found out. They develop coping strategies to hide their difficulties. Some adults will have developed negative strategies such as quitting their job rather than risking the humiliation of their employment being terminated because their DCD makes it difficult for them to keep up with work demands.

Adults with social skill difficulties may live in fear of revealing social inadequacies. For example, adults who have trouble understanding humour may pretend to laugh at a joke even though they don't understand it. They may also hide their social difficulties by appearing to be shy and withdrawn. On the other hand, the more hyperactive adults may cover up their attention difficulties by being outgoing and extravert to entertain people.

Failure

For most people, anxiety about failing is what motivates them to succeed, but for people with DCD, this anxiety can be paralysing. Fear of failure may prevent them from making the most of new opportunities. It might inhibit them from participating in social activities, taking on a new job or enrolling in an adult education course.

One positive characteristic that often helps adults overcome their fear of failure is an ability to develop innovative strategies to manage situations and to problem-solve. These strategies are often attributed to the 'learned creativity' that many adults develop in order to cope with the everyday demands in their lives (Gerber et al., 1992).

Ridicule

Adults with DCD frequently fear the ridicule of others. Sadly, these fears often develop after the individual has been routinely ridiculed by teachers, classmates or even family members. The most demoralizing of these criticisms usually relates to a perceived lack of intelligence or unfair judgments about the person's motivation or ability to succeed. For example, comments such as 'you'll never amount to anything', 'you could do it if you only tried harder'.

Rejection

Adults with DCD frequently fear rejection if they are not seen to be as capable as others. They may also fear that any social skill deficits will preclude them from building meaningful relationships with others and lead to social rejection. Prior experiences of rejection will likely intensify this sense of fear.

One adult with DCD reported:

> It took me 37 years to get a diagnosis. I was admitted to a 'mental' hospital 3 days before my 21st birthday due to a breakdown. I became agoraphobic and suffered severe depression. My self-esteem was as low as I have ever known it.

Sensitivity and modulation

Adults with DCD are often overwhelmed by too much environmental stimuli (e.g. background noise, more than one person talking at a time, side conversations, reading and listening at the same time). Some individuals with DCD have specific sensitivities to their environment, such as certain fabrics they cannot wear, foods they cannot tolerate, etc.

They may also see themselves as more emotionally sensitive than other people. Fortunately, most adults have learned to handle their emotional sensitivity to avoid becoming overwhelmed or engaging in negative social interactions. Nevertheless, some adults may be so deeply affected that they become depressed or suffer from anxiety. Emotional wounds from childhood and youth may cause heightened emotional responses to rejection. In turn, social anxiety and social phobia may result.

Adjusting to change

Change is scary for everyone, but for people with DCD and other neuro-developmental disorders, change may be particularly difficult. For example, some adults will have trouble moving from one work task to another without completely finishing the first task before moving on to the next one. They are frequently described as inflexible when it comes to considering another person's viewpoint or a different way of doing something.

Adjustment to change is not easy because change brings the unexpected. In general, those with DCD are less prepared for the unexpected. The unexpected may bring new learning hurdles, new job demands or new social challenges. To avoid the tendency to blame the person for their lack of flexibility, it is important to understand the neurological basis for this difficulty with adjusting to change. However, through social skills practice, adults with DCD can improve their ability to tolerate change.

Social skills and relationships

Difficulties with social interaction have been identified as a common characteristic in conditions such as DCD (Hazel and Schumaker, 1988; Mellard and Hazel, 1992). Given that one's general life satisfaction and adjustment as an adult is seen as largely dependent on one's social competence, researchers suggest that those whose difficulties affect skills relating to social realms are more than likely to be dissatisfied as adults. White's (1992) review of literature found that most adults with DCD-related conditions were single, living with parents or relatives and they participated in fewer recreational, social and community activities than those without. They were also found to have fewer friends and were much less satisfied with their family relationships.

Smith (1987) describes characteristics relevant to those who lack social skills:

- difficulty in turn-taking in conversation – tendency to interrupt frequently;
- lack of emotional/facial expression;
- poor eye contact;
- violation of territorial space (sit or stand too close);
- failure to follow a conversation;
- respond impulsively;
- share information that is inappropriately intimate;
- difficulty taking another's perspective;
- responding defensively;
- disorganized;
- tendency to blame others for mistakes and failures;
- rambling or straying off topic frequently during conversation.

> I speak too loudly but at other times speak too softly. I am bad at making eye contact. I think more quickly than my brain can process the thoughts and end up blurting things out inappropriately. I frequently interrupt others without realizing it, but resist all the appropriate signs and go on talking. In company people are too polite to point this out but it's interesting that people do not seek me out for second and subsequent conversations. It is not uncommon for me to fail to dress properly and leave zips and buttons undone or misaligned. (Andrew Hatton, DANDA Issue 2, 2004)

Relationships

Relationships have a significant effect on the development of health and well-being of individuals. Most people want to be liked and tend to feel happy when they are part of a group or feel they have friends and are considered to be a friend by others. Many adults with DCD find it difficult to make and maintain friendships; therefore entering into more intimate relationships can also be difficult. The success of forming relationships is based upon social skills as previously discussed. A good self-image is also important.

Self-concept and self-image

- Self-concept is how see ourselves.
- Self-image is how we value ourselves. It results from the way in which we have been treated by others. Positive relationships tend to encourage a positive self-image and feelings of confidence and self-belief. Negative relationships can lead to seeing ourselves as being of little value and having no confidence and no self-belief. This is because most of self-image is formed by the way others make us feel.

Both self-concept and self-image are influenced by the relationships we have throughout our lives (see Table 7.1).

Table 7.1 Influence of relationships on self-concept and self-image

Positive relationships	Negative relationships
Confidence in making own decisions	No confidence in own abilities
Confidence in abilities	Not being able to be part of a group
Feeling liked by others	Self-doubt
High self-esteem	Feeling isolated
Able to make friendships	Feeling of worthlessness/low self-esteem
Feeling of belonging	Difficulty in relating to others/unable to form long-term relationships
Security	Insecurity

There are alternative methods for overcoming barriers and encouraging communication:

- letter – pen pals;
- telephone;
- camcorder/video;
- emails;

* Internet chat rooms/webcams;
* texting.

Developing social skills

To enable adults with DCD, many need support and guidance in the adjustment and modulation of their social skills. The following may be considered in intervention approaches:

* effective communication skills, negotiation and conflict resolution;
* how to accept and give praise and criticism;
* identifying and adjusting communication styles and building relationships to effect support;
* assertive communication and interpersonal problem-solving.

DCD and the need for fitness

The importance of fitness to our general health and well-being is well documented, with increasing worldwide concern about lack of exercise. From childhood, children with DCD are noted to be less fit and physically competent than co-ordinated children. The results of poor co-ordination and the accompanying feelings of inadequacy are constantly reinforced in school (playground/PE and games). The long-term consequence is reduced motivation to participate in physical activities, few interactions with the environment and consequently fewer opportunities to develop proficient motor skills and fitness. From the limited longitudinal studies, the same appears to apply in adolescents and adults (Cermak and Larkin, 2002).

Inefficient patterns of movement and mechanical inefficiency can require higher demands of energy. As a consequence both children and adults with DCD can fatigue much earlier that better co-ordinated people (O'Beirne et al., 1994). Fatigue reduces the ability to contribute joyfully and participate enthusiastically in many daily activities. Early fatigue accompanying the low levels of fitness contributes to discomfort and lower levels of exercise tolerance (Cermak and Larkin, 2002).

Individuals with DCD commonly have low muscle strength (Casperson et al., 1985). Poor muscle strength in the body may indicate a potential to develop musculoskeletal problems such as low back pain.

For those with limited flexibility gentle and regular stretching is helpful. Activities to help:

* yoga
* Pilates

- Tai Chi
- Alexander technique
- swimming/aqua aerobics
- horse riding
- canoeing
- abseiling/indoor climbing
- gym clubs
- country dancing
- badminton
- rambling/walking

Fitness can be improved. Individuals need to participate in regular, preferably daily, physical activity. However, as individuals with DCD find movement difficult and not enjoyable, more structure, direction and alternative activities are necessary. See Appendix VII for useful contacts and organizations.

- Exercises that increase range of movement in shoulders and arms will also prevent stiffness and make dressing and grooming easier.
- Integrate activities that will improve general fitness into lifestyle; walk to the shops, walk up stairs rather than using the lift in shops, go for a short walk regularly, go swimming once a week/fortnight.
- Choose non-competitive sports and evening classes that will promote more control over goals and pace of work.

On a lighter note . . . .

> After trying on my bikini for my holiday, I found I could do with toning up. I decided to get a fitness ball and video. Unfortunately because I get confused on opening and closing my Venetian blinds, the neighbours now get a good view of my uncoordinated attempts at following the movements on the video and me falling off the exercise ball. (Adult with DCD)

Hobbies and interests

Loneliness or lack of anything interesting to do during the day may exacerbate any existing feelings of low self-worth. It is therefore important for individuals with DCD to have interests and hobbies and participate in daily occupations that make them feel valued.

In order to support adults with DCD in developing leisure pursuits an interest index could be carried out (see Figure 7.1).

Key to good practice
- Get to know the individual's interests and needs
- Work at the individual's pace

- Don't impose views about suitability or appropriateness
- Be realistic about what is available
- Keep information accurate and up-to-date

It may be useful to keep a 'who', 'what', 'where' list of local facilities and resources. An example is given in Figure 7.3.

Take care not to provide the individual with unrealistic expectations about services and facilities available to them in the local area. It may be helpful to have a regular list of activities and resources which may be of interest. Table 7.2 considers the benefits of a selection of hobbies and interests which may be helpful to an individual with DCD.

Table 7.2 Benefits of hobbies and interests

Activity	Promotes
Social Events within local community Visits to places of interest	Health and well-being Prevents isolation Emotional and social needs Interests and stimulation
Intellectual Word games Chess Using the internet Evening classes	Verbal skills Stimulates thought processes and problem-solving Orientation Maintains intellect
Spiritual Attending religious services	Meets need for pastoral/spiritual care Comfort Maintains religious beliefs Mood and self-esteem Opportunities for socialization
Speciality Yoga	Improves health and fitness Motivation Motor control and co-ordination Attention span and concentration
Creative Art/craft Creative writing Music	Cognitive skills Self-esteem Motor control and co-ordination Social
Physical Walking Swimming Golf	Cardiovascular fitness Tones muscles Feeling of well-being

Activity	Don't do/ not interested	Don't do/ would like to do	Do at least once a week	Do at least three times a week
Movies				
Visit/entertain relatives				
Use PC/Internet				
Meet with friends				
Social clubs/groups				
Crafts				
Cooking				
Painting				
Gardening				
Reading				
Theatre/concerts				
Swimming or other fitness activity				

Figure 7.1 Example of Interest Index

Table 7.3 Services and facilities checklist

What	Who	Where
Holidays	Specialist travel companies	Internet
Sports and Leisure	Winged Fellowship	Travel Agents
Cinemas	Solo Holidays	Library
	Leisure Services department	Internet
	Riding for the Disabled	Local paper
	Outward Bound trust	What's On
	Leisure Services department	Guide
		Internet
		Library
		Local Paper

Home services

Depending on the individual's circumstances, they may wish to take advantage of services that can be supplied to them in their own home setting rather than having to travel. There may also be services that can provide off-site facilities such as mobile libraries.

Travelling to services

Some individuals may prefer to use local bus services or may be able to drive. In some localities it may be possible for individuals to obtain concessionary travel rates for public transport. Alternatively they could take a taxi, or travel with a friend/family member.

Barriers to accessing activities

Environmental

- Literacy – reading information or filling in forms
- Orientation skills within a building, e.g. finding rooms within a large complex
- Transport
- Threatening location

Communication

- Lack of information
- Unhelpful staff at facility
- Communication skills of the individual

Psychological

- Fear and anxiety
- Unfamiliarity
- Unwillingness to accept help
- Lack of confidence

Getting around

Some adults with DCD have poor orientation skills. It may be necessary to practise excursions and visits in advance several times to build up confidence and security in orientation. Visual markers such as landmarks will help reinforce the route.

If using a bus the use of bus passes can reduce the need to find the correct money.

Driving

Learning to drive a car or motorcycle can prove to be difficult for young people and adults with DCD. It may take them considerably longer to learn to drive as there are a number of skills to master and co-ordinate at the same time, e.g. concentrating, judging distance, steering and using both hands and feet at the same time while changing gears. In addition, having to remember the sequence of the steps necessary to successfully carry out required manoeuvres adds to the difficulty.

Choosing a driving instructor

- Find a driving school that has taught people with disabilities before and which has an understanding of specific learning difficulties.
- The British School of Motoring (BSM) offers special courses that cater for the needs of people with specific learning difficulties. They also have a CD programme called MAP that can help with some of the skills required for driving. Some BSM branches have driving simulators with geared cars, which enable people to build up their confidence before driving on the open road.
- Within the UK are a number of specialist assessment centres that can assess driving skills in a safe environment in order to establish the learner driver's abilities. Details of such centres can be obtained from the Department of Transport's Mobility Advice and Information Service (MAVIS) – see Appendix IV.

Applying for a driving test

- It may be possible to request extra time to complete the theory/written section. Information about concessions on the theory test is available from Drive Safe, Driving Standards Agency Special Needs Team – see Appendix IV.
- A range of books, videos and CD ROMs to assist with the preparation of theory/written tests is commercially available from good newsagents, libraries and bookshops.

Driving tips

- Individuals with DCD often find it easier to learn in an automatic car. This reduces the number of tasks to be carried out at the same time and requires less co-ordination.
- Mark one side of the steering wheel with a sticker as a visual aide-memoire to remember which side is left and which is right.
- Plan and prepare for journeys in advance. Write directions down and clip them to the dashboard where they can be easily seen.
- GPS (satellite navigational systems) are now commonly available accessories that can save the need for map reading.
- Fit reversing indicators that sound as the car approaches an object in close proximity.

A driver's tale

On a trip to Brittany I was asked to look at the map and tell the driver what turnings to take. 'Are you sure I said, I am rubbish at things like that.' So we pulled over and the driver showed me where we were and what to follow. So I thought I had got the hang of it. I followed the road with my finger, passing all the points that were coming up and it looked good. We finally took a stop and realized that we had driven 2 hours in the wrong direction. We left England at 6 am and were due to arrive at our destination at 5 pm in time for tea. We turned up at 11 pm . . . and the car broke down!!

Summary

Numerous studies have examined the social, emotional and behavioural problems associated with motor difficulties, leading to growing evidence that the lack of movement skill may have damaging consequences for social and psychological development.

Studies of adolescents with DCD have shown consistently lower health-related and skill-related fitness levels than the average individuals. Adult studies are not yet available but a similar picture is predicted. The low levels of fitness can contribute to early fatigue and limit motor skill development.

Many adults with DCD engage less in recreational activities and tend to remain single and living at home with parents or relatives.

In view of the likelihood of developing social and emotional difficulties, the importance of leisure and a healthy lifestyle for adults with DCD is significant. Unfortunately motivational factors based on previous experiences weigh heavily. However, for those who have been able to find solace in a leisure pursuit, they have often been able to reveal strengths previously unrecognized.

CHAPTER 8
The adult at home

Activities of daily living

Taber (1997) defines 'activities of daily living' as tasks that enable individuals to meet basic needs. Five task areas are identified as: personal care, family responsibilities, work or school, recreation and socialization.

Living completely independently is a highly complex skill and in the normal course of development, skills are gradually acquired through childhood and adolescence. The process usually culminates with each individual leaving the parental home to live a separate life. Independence relates in part to being able to work and support one's self and family, having the freedom to go where one wants and when, and the privacy and ability to look after oneself (Turner, 1987). If this is compromised in any way then self-esteem can be affected as individuals may not value themselves or expect others to do so.

For adolescents who were diagnosed with mild DCD at a younger age, the research suggests that they may not have many functional problems. However, for those with moderate to severe DCD, difficulties may continue to manifest later on (Cantell et al., 1994). Coping with DCD in adult life is not just about work, but also what happens in and around the home. Depending on severity, even the simplest of tasks normally taken for granted can seem daunting. Preparing for and clearing up after meals can take twice as long, since those with DCD find tasks such as peeling, chopping, stirring, opening cans, cartons and jars difficult. Many forget that they have put something on the stove, leading to near-miss fires and certainly ruined pots and pans. Operating and using electrical equipment such as washing machines can prove to be an ordeal. Evidence suggests that motor problems may primarily remain in areas involving manual dexterity (Geuze and Borger, 1993).

Aspects of activities of daily living that need to be developed in the adult with DCD are:

• personal skills – needed to establish and maintain a network of appropriate and meaningful relationships;
• home management skills – the technical and theoretical know-how to live safely, comfortably and healthily;
• self-reliance – what the individual needs to organize and maintain the resources they need.

One adult with DCD reported:

> Nothing came naturally to me, even things like cooking and ironing had to be broken down into small steps for me to follow and that was a tremendous effort. (Eckersley, 2004, p. 55)

Another adult reported:

> At home I can't do things like changing the duvet and cooking. I keep life as simple as possible: I buy clothes that don't need ironing. I keep my hair in a style that is easy to manage so I don't have to fiddle about with clips or bands. I also keep my make-up to a minimum.

To an adult with DCD, the ability to perform these tasks may mean the difference between being independent and dependent. Supporting and enabling an adult with DCD at home in everyday living activities can be:

• Through training the individual in developing certain techniques for task completion;
• Assisting the individual by using an easier or alternative method, or utilizing a small aid or piece of equipment;
• Finding solutions to practical problems.

Often simple and straightforward ideas can make life easier. Table 8.1 lists some practical suggestions and strategies that people have found useful. An example of a life skills questionnaire (Figure 8.2) can also be found at the end of the chapter.

Table 8.1 Areas of difficulty, functional implications and strategies

Area of difficulty	Functional implications	Strategies
Co-ordination	Poor manual dexterity can lead to difficulties with preparing meals, operating domestic	• Use longer-handled tools e.g. a dustpan with a long handle is easier to use than traditional ones. • Choose easy-care clothes and bedlinen to reduce need for ironing.

Table 8.1 continued

Area of difficulty	Functional implications	Strategies
Co-ordination (contd)	equipment, unscrewing things, opening doors and locks and fiddly or intricate tasks. Frequently drop things and unintentionally break things. Clumsy gait and movement result in tripping or bumping into furniture etc.	• Patterned fabrics mask stains better than plain ones. • Use washing machine nets to keep small items together. • Sock clips help keep socks together in matched pairs. • Buy cordless kettles and irons as they are easier to use. • Use Dycem or a damp dishcloth under plates, dishes and pans to stop them moving. • Make use of labour-saving devices such as electric tin openers, toasters, cordless kettles, talking scales. • Microwave ovens are easier to use than traditional ovens.

Organization and time management	Difficulty organizing household routines e.g. plan, shop, prepare a meal and clean up afterwards.
	
	Difficulty organizing accommodation/ home, belongings and keeping them clean.
	
	Frequently being late for work, appointments and public transport can have a negative effect on friendships and other relationships.
	
	Difficulty finding the way around new places, towns and buildings.
		• Establish daily routines and then keep to them.
		• Use a personal organizer or diary to record appointments:
		  – Mark each day to clearly identify a.m./p.m.
		  – Block out periods of time that are routine i.e. grocery shopping, go to the bank etc.
		  – Mark the current page by holding previous pages to the front cover with an elastic band.
		  – Use highlighters to mark important appointments.
		• Use a notice board/pin board to pin up reminders and 'To do' job list.
		• Use a Dictaphone, talking pen, mini-microphone, reminder key rings, or a mini notepad to record things that have been forgotten.
		• Use labelled filing trays for storing mail and bills to be paid. Check them weekly.
		• Read instructions, read out loud as if giving the instruction, then try picturing the actions. Use mental rehearsal or a personal running

Table 8.1 continued

Area of difficulty	Functional implications	Strategies
Organization and time management (contd)		commentary to help remember the sequence of tasks. • Prepare instructions in advance. Write them out on small cards, numbered in sequence, using key words or diagrams. • Ask friends/family to demonstrate how something needs to be done rather than just be given instructions. • Print own name/calling cards with address and telephone numbers on. • Use a kitchen timer or watch with a buzzer to help with awareness of time.
Managing finances	Difficulty understanding figures and budgeting. Even though they may understand the benefits of saving and of budgeting, they may need help identifying and setting up practical strategies and methods. Establishing level of help and support: Consider the reasons why the individual needs help. Is it because: • They are specifically unable to make payments. • They are confused and forget to make payments. • They are unsure what payments they need to make. • They are unlikely to be able to motivate or organize themselves to make payments on time. • They do not recognize the importance of making the payment.	• Use labelled filing trays for storing mail to be dealt with and bills to be paid. Check them weekly. • Use a lever arch file with clearly labelled plastic polypockets in it for storing paid bills and important information. • Create a shopping list template for items bought regularly i.e. cheese, eggs and bread. Before going shopping add additional items to the list that are required that day. • Shopping on the Internet can be easier than physically going shopping. *Strategies for managing money:* • Direct Debits • Budget Accounts • Arrange for income to be paid directly into bank account Most banks will be able to advise with regard to services that can help manage money. *Dealing with debt:* Enlist the help of experienced debt counsellors. These are available through Citizens Advice Bureaux, Welfare Rights Advice Centres and local Money Advice Centres.

Table 8.1 continued

Area of difficulty	Functional implications	Strategies
Personal care and hygiene		
Dressing	Managing buttons, zips and other fastenings Matching garments Orientation of garments	• Buy clothes with few or no fastenings, such as trousers/shorts with elasticated waists and t-shirts/polo shirts. • Use alternatives to traditional fastenings – poppers and Velcro are easier to operate than laces, small buttons and zips. • Peg shoes together to help find them in the wardrobe. • Look for visual clues such as logos, seams and labels that indicate the garment's front/back, inside/outside. • Organize clothes by colour in the wardrobe. • Use drawer tidies to store socks and underwear. • Use see-through boxes for shoes.
Hair Eyebrows	Styling hair	• Have a hairstyle that is easy to keep - a style that can be almost dried with 'rough drying' first and then finished off with some gel to keep it in place is easy to manage. • Using a long-handled hairbrush and/or comb can help reach the back of the hair. • Invest in regular visits to the hairdresser/barber. *Eyebrows:* Invest in regular appointments with the local beautician.
Teeth	Holding and manipulating the toothbrush around the inside of the mouth	• Use an electric toothbrush. • Regular check-ups at the dentist. • Use an anti-bacterial mouthwash. For fresh breath when out, try using sugar-free chewing-gum.
Shaving	Holding and manipulating the shaver around the contours of the face	*Males:* • Use electric shavers. • Pick a shaver that has a built-in safety guard.

Table 8.1 continued

Area of difficulty	Functional implications	Strategies
Personal care and hygiene Shaving (contd)	and removing facial hair	• A good magnifying mirror will make it easier to remove facial hair. *Females:* • Use hair-removing cream instead of shaving legs and underarms. Having a leg wax by someone else may also solve the problem.
Menstruation	Poor sense of time may lead to forgetting to change pad or tampon Manipulating pads or tampons	• Stick-on pads (without side panels or 'wings') are easier to place. • Some ladies may need a reminder to change their pads/tampons. A watch or mobile phone with a timer set to go off every few hours can help.
Bathing Showering Toileting	Cleansing self after passing a motion Reaching body parts to wash Safely getting in and out of bath/shower	• Using moist toilet wipes after using the toilet can help with cleansing. • A bath mat placed in the bath/shower will stop slipping. • Use long-handled sponges. • Use a soap mitt (where the soap is inserted inside a small pocket (palm side)). • Use a towelling robe rather than a towel.
Contraception	Forgetting to take tablets	• A buzzer reminder or a talking alarm clock can be used as a reminder to take the pill each morning upon wakening. If it is part of a sequence of other activities, like teeth cleaning, it is less likely to be forgotten. • There is an injectable form of contraception that needs to be given every 12 weeks. The GP or family planning clinic should be consulted about this.
Eating and drinking	Managing cutlery	• Don't fill cups too full. • Using cups with larger handles provides a better grip.

Table 8.1 continued

Area of difficulty	Functional implications	Strategies
Personal care and hygiene		
Eating and drinking (contd)	Spilling drinks/liquids	• A kettle tipper may help make pouring easier and safer. • Avoid choosing foods such as spaghetti and chicken on the bone when dining out.
Sleep	Some adults with DCD may have problems with sleeping. Should the individual have continued difficulties in this area with signs of early morning wakening and significant difficulties getting off to sleep, then their GP should be consulted.	• Consider if the bedroom environment is too noisy. • The bedroom may be too light. Is the temperature too high or low? • Is the bedroom too dark? • Is the bed comfortable? Is it an old one? • Is there an allergy to the pillows or the duvet?

Other jobs around the house

In the garden

Gardening can be very therapeutic. It gives a sense of reward and satisfaction whether flowers or vegetables are grown.

However, the need to organize jobs in the garden as the seasons change can be daunting, as can weeding and using the plethora of tools to do the job.

Tips

• Use ergonomic tools – lightweight tools, tools with large soft handles, use extension handles where necessary to save reaching and over-stretching. Use long-handled tools to avoid stooping and poor posture when working.
• Pave, patio and gravel where possible to save cutting the lawn and doing the edges.
• Use mulches, wood bark on beds to save weeding.

- Use container pots, raised beds, hanging baskets to add colour but save on bending.
- Use hardy plants and perennials to provide all year round colour.
- Choose flowers that can survive some neglect, e.g. don't need too much watering.
- Use an irrigation watering system on a timer.
- Make gardening a family task.

DIY

A DCD adult may never master skills requiring co-ordination such as performing simple DIY jobs, repairing or mending things, because they may be unable to use tools or implements. They are thus unable to perform simple and basic tasks that most people take for granted. This means that the individual has many disadvantages not envisaged by other people, and as such may be forced to pay for simple jobs to be done. (Colley, 2000, p. 65)

The simplest of chores such as screwing a screw into the wall, can be difficult for the adult with DCD. Needless to say the job of putting together a flat pack piece of furniture daunts the majority of the population.

Tips

- Emulsion walls rather than use wallpaper – use rollers rather than brushes. Use long-handled brushes to save climbing ladders.
- If replacing windows, guttering and fascias, consider UPVC to save repainting.
- Use magnetic battery-operated screwdrivers – save on losing those little screws.
- Use wood glues and adhesives rather than drills if appropriate.
- Organize maintenance jobs to be routinely done.

The parent with DCD

Difficulties in the ability to perform everyday tasks and activities often subsequently result in an inability to fully participate in appropriate social roles (WHO, 1997).

The roles of father, husband, wife, mother, add new dimensions of complexity to the daily life of someone with DCD. In society women tend to bear the responsibility for maintaining the household and raising the children. The man tends to be responsible for the more physical aspects of the home as well as share in some of the other jobs needed to run the household smoothly.

Some individuals feel totally overwhelmed at the sheer number of tasks in the home. It may be too difficult for them to break the tasks down and prioritize them. This puts them under a lot of stress and they may 'blow a fuse' at the slightest thing, especially if they are trying to do a few things at the same time, e.g. prepare a meal and answer the door. This often leads to the children being punished or reprimanded unfairly, or big arguments break out.

This does not mean to say that this does not happen in most households as parenting is an ever-changing role that challenges most adults. However, the adult with DCD invariably needs to rely on the strengths of the partner as well as the children to support them in everyday tasks.

Organizing the family home and schedules can be difficult. Creating family routines can make everyday activities more manageable. For example, mornings and early evenings can be stressful. These are times when homework, sports or music lessons might take place creating more demands on adult time. Families can be assisted in developing strategies, such as using a calendar with all the family's important dates, colour-coding each family member for the various appointments. Holding family meetings every Sunday to discuss what is happening in the coming week is also helpful. Designating certain chores to various family members can also help to reduce unnecessary pressure and stress.

Being the spouse/partner of an adult with DCD

Maintaining long-lasting and satisfying relationships with a spouse or partner with DCD can be challenging. Some of the behaviours may annoy the partner who might then criticize leaving a sense of dissatisfaction in the relationship.

Sometimes marriages or partnerships with an adult with DCD work well. The partner may provide stability, structure and organizational skills. When each partner has an insight into their unique strengths and weaknesses, they can learn from each other in a dynamic way and not allow their roles to become too rigid.

Dependency can be an issue and this may cause conflict.

Occasionally individuals with DCD marry or live together. They may find that at last they have found someone on their own 'wavelength'. However, when couples enter into the complex family demands, they may need outside help to 'stabilize' their lives.

In building stronger relationships the partner needs to:

• understand and appreciate how DCD affects behaviour and the ability to communicate;
• understand that some tasks may take longer to do than other people;

- use strategies to help their partner with DCD e.g. write down instructions for jobs that need doing;
- agree a trade-off in household chores;
- not expect partners to read each other's minds;
- avoid personal criticism – 'you're messy all the time', 'you never listen to me'.

Benefits and financial support

Individuals with DCD may be eligible for benefits (see Figure 8.1). Sources of information for benefits and allowances are extremely varied throughout the country. The most comprehensive advice and information is available at centres such as Citizens Advice Bureaux. They also have a website and telephone helpline. The Benefits Agency also provides a helpline; however, this only relates to state benefits. An example of a financial affairs checklist is illustrated in Figure 8.3.

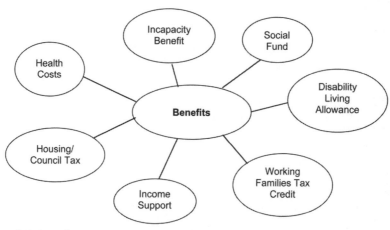

Figure 8.1 Benefits.

Summary

It appears that, across their lifespan, individuals with DCD continue to experience difficulties with activities of daily living. As the young person grows, the expectations increase and so do the levels of frustration when attempting many activities. Those with mild difficulties often accommodate to them and eventually master skills, but those with moderate to severe difficulties continue to experience difficulties across a range of skills and tasks. Adaptations and practical strategies can increase the success of the individual leading to success within the home and daily life.

Name…….…..……………………………………….DOB…………..…………….Date…………….

Rate your level of skill/ability to each question:

1.   No skill/unable to
2.   Attempt task but require physical support
3.   Can complete part of task independently but require support
4.   Require verbal prompts/reminders to complete task
5.   Able to competently complete task with confidence

PRACTICAL SKILLS	RATING	COMMENT
Self-care: Getting up in the morning – bath/shower		
Personal hygiene (brushing teeth, shaving, feminine hygiene, make-up etc.)		
Getting organized for the day		
Laundry – washing i.e. sorting and knowledge of fabrics etc.		
– ironing		
Opening cartons, packets and cans		
Making a simple meal – including vegetable preparation and cooking more than one item		
Making a snack – using a grill/toaster		
Keeping room/house tidy		
Using household appliances		
Getting around buildings/towns – finding places and using maps		
Ability to use buses, trains, taxis – reading timetables		
Managing money – checking change		
– using a bank account		
– using a plastic card		
– using cash machines		
– writing cheques		
Filling in forms		
Driving – theory test, learning		
Dealing with correspondence/paying bills		
Gardening		
Leisure		
DIY – fixing/repairs		
What to do in an emergency – medical or appliance breakdown		
Pet care – caring for others		
Taking medication – simple first aid		
Planning for events e.g. holidays, Christmas, BBQs		
SOCIAL SKILLS	RATING	COMMENT
Ability to get on with others/conversational skills		
Reading other people's body language		
Coping with others' requests/saying 'no'		
Handling criticism/ put-down comments		
Accepting praise		
Keeping appointments/time-keeping		

Figure 8.2 Life Skills Questionnaire – Adult.

Income/Expenditure Budget Chart			
INCOME	Weekly	Monthly	Yearly
Salary/wage			
Other			
Pension			
Job Seekers' Allowance			
Income Support			
Housing Benefit			
Other Benefits			
Interest on Savings			
TOTAL			
EXPENDITURE			
Mortgage or Rent			
Loans/Credit cards			
Council Tax			
Water Rates			
Ground Rent			
Repairs and Maintenance			
Contents Insurance			
Gas			
Electricity			
Telephone			
Food			
Clothing			
TV Rental/Licence			
Prescriptions			
Health Insurance			
Public Transport			
Holidays			
Pension Contributions			
Regular Savings			
Maintenance Payments			
TOTAL			
FINANCIAL POSITION			
Total Income			
Total Expenditure			
Financial Position			

Figure 8.3 Administering financial affairs checklist.

The adult learner

Useful websites

Education

www.canterbury.ac.uk/xplanatory/xplan.htm
Useful site with over 600 pages of information dealing with special needs, access and inclusion.

Teachability

Audit materials for use with academic departments, available from www.teachability.strath.ac.uk

SENDA Compliance in Higher Education – a guidance tool for accessible practice within the framework of teaching and learning. Available at www.plymouth.ac.uk/disability

Accessible curricula: good practice for all

For general information about good practice in learning and teaching for disabled students. Available on www.techdis.ac.uk

Code of Practice for the Assurance of Academic Quality and Standards in Higher Education. Section 3: Students with Disabilities

Available from The Quality Assurance Agency for Higher Education. www.qaa.ac.uk

Electronic learning

For information on making electronic material accessible. www.techdis.ac.uk

Study skills

Bangor University website which has information about study skills techniques and study aids.
www.dyslexia.bangor.ac.uk

Essay writing tips for HE students
www.brad.ac.uk/acad/civeng/skills/essays.htm

Legislation and guidance

The Disability Rights Commission
For organizations that offer disability equality training see
www.drc-gb.org

For information on legal responsibilities towards disabled students and applicants under the Disability Discrimination Act see:
Code of Practice for Providers of Post-16 Education and Related Services, available from the Disability Rights Commission Helpline

or contact:

The Disability Rights Commission Helpline
DRC Helpline
Freepost
MID 02164
Stratford upon Avon CV37 9BR
Tel: 08457 622 633
Textphone: 08457 622 644
Fax: 08457 778 878
Email: enquiry@drc-gb.org
www.drc-gb.org

Skill: National Bureau for Students with Disabilities
Information Service
Chapter House
18–20 Crucifix Lane
London SE1 3JW
Tel: 0800 328 5050
Textphone: 0800 068 2422
Email: info@skill.org.uk
www.skill.org.uk

Advisory Centre for Education
Guidance and interpretation of the law in relation to SEN.
www.ace-ed.org.uk

CSIE (Centre for Studies on Inclusive Education)
Lists the Salamanca statement on SEN by UNESCO as well as other links
dealing with inclusion.
www.inclusion_uwe.ac.uk/csie/csiehome.htm

Useful organizations

Learn Direct
Helpline: 0800 100 900
Course information: 0800 101 901
www.learndirect.co.uk
Courses available through the Internet.

Open University
Tel: 0870 330 087 (for regional centre)
Email: generalrequests@open.ac.uk
www.open.ac.uk
The OU provides supported distance learning in a range of subjects. No
formal entrance qualifications required.

Communication and Learning Skills Centre (CALSC)
131 Himefield Park
Sutton
Surrey, SM1 2DY
Tel: 020 8642 4663
Email: info@calsc.co.uk
Produces a range of learning aids such as student organizer packs.

Basic Skills Agency (BSA)
Commonwealth House
1–19 New Oxford Street
London WC1A 1NU
Tel: 020 7405 4017
Fax: 020 7440 6626
Publications order line: 0870 600 2400
Email: enquiries@basic-skills.co.uk
www.basic-skills.co.uk
This organization operates a free national telephone referral service to
help individuals find the nearest centre. It is for those over 16 years and

no longer in full-time education and offers help with literacy, basic maths and linked skills such as computing.

Skill: National Bureau for Students with Disabilities
4th Floor, Chapter House
18–20 Crucifix Lane
London SE1 3JW
Tel: 020 7450 0620
Fax: 020 7450 0650
Information Service tel: 0800 328 5050 (Mon–Thurs, 13.30–16.30)
Email: info@skill.org.uk
www.skill.org.uk
Has information about specific forms of support that may be helpful for students in further or higher education who have a specific learning difficulty.

Department for Education and Skills (DfES)
Sanctuary Buildings
Great Smith Street
London SW1 3BT
Tel: 0870 000 2288
Email: info@dfes.gsi.gov.uk
www.dfes.gov.uk
Centre for SEN website www.dfes.gov.uk/sen
Publications order line tel: 0845 602 2260

Useful booklets available free from the DfES, tel: 0800 731 9133

Bridging the Gap – A Guide to Disability Student Allowances (DSAs) in Higher Education
Financial Support for Higher Education Students

National Association for Special Educational Needs (NASEN)
4–5 Amber Business Village
Amber Close
Amington
Tamworth
Staffordshire B77 4RP
Tel: 01827 311 500
www.nasen.org.uk

Useful books/resources

Use Your Head
Tony Buzan
BBC Books, 2003

The Secrets of Successful Students: Super Speed Study Skills
Michael Tipper
Lucky Duck Publishing Ltd, 2002

In the Mind's Eye
TG West
Buffalo, New York, Prometheus Books, 1997

Student Organizer Pack
JE Mitchell
Communication and Learning Skills Centre
www.calsc.co.uk

Master It Faster
C Rose
Accelerated Learning, 1999

Assistive technology and ICT

Assistive technology

www.attainmentcompany.com

- Time Pad – five recorded messages can be activated by setting a timer for predetermined times. Helps with remembering a sequence of activities.
- Step Pad – records and plays back messages one step at a time. Helpful for those who have difficulty remembering a sequence of steps.
- Motionpad – designed to be hung on a wall or door. It automatically plays either a message or a chime (indicating there is a message) when someone enters the room or area.
- Memo Talker – this is a single 20-second message device.
- Talking Key Chain Clock – for those who understand time better when given as an auditory cue.
- Voice recording pen – a ballpoint pen that can also record speech for instant playback. Up to 10 seconds of recording time.

Reading Pen

Designed for those who require support with reading. It is ideal to help with reading words the user cannot spell, pronounce or comprehend. Available from Iansyst (see below).

Programs

Kurzweil 3000
Offers a combined scanning and reading application that allows printed script to be converted into audio feedback. It also has a number of study skills tools such as audible spell-checking, word prediction, dictionaries. Available from IANSYST (see below).

Read 7 Write Gold
This is a completely integrated system that offers speech feedback, word prediction and scanning. It includes a phonetic spell-checker, word prediction and talking calculator. Available from IANSYST (see below).

Dragon Naturally Speaking
Enables the user to dictate continuously into many applications including Microsoft Word and Excel. It is a tool for those who find getting their thoughts on to paper difficult but can articulate their ideas.

Franklin Pocket Dictionary/Thesaurus
A small portable UK dictionary and thesaurus with phonic spell-checker.

Inspiration
A powerful visual learning tool to inspire users to develop their ideas while planning and structuring workflow. Interactive diagrams, charts and reports help organize and prioritize concepts and information. Available from The Dyscovery Centre (see below).

Mindful
A simple planning tool for creating on-screen mind maps and concept maps available from The Dyscovery Centre (see below).

SpeakOUT
Is a text-to-speech program to support reading and writing difficulties. Available from The Dyscovery Centre (see below).

Post IT
A simple and easy 'post it' note type aide-memoire that sits on the computer desktop. It can also be used to devise timetables and planners. Available from The Dyscovery Centre (see below).

Watch Minder
This is a regular watch with added functions. The watch can be programmed to go off at set times to act as an external reminder or prompter to complete tasks. Available from The Dyscovery Centre (see below).

Useful organizations

AbilityNet
PO Box 94
Warwick CV34 5WS
Tel: 01926 312847
National Freephone 0800 269 545

www.abilitynet.org.uk
Provides an information and advice service on computing for disabled people, including computing at work, individual assessments, training and consultancy.

AbilityNet Technical Centre
Suite 1 Malvern Gate
Bromwich Road
Worcester WR2 4BN
Tel: 01905 420520
Can supply computers and computer solutions (following assessment) with emphasis on individual need and support.

Ace Centre
92 Windmill Road
Headington
Oxford OX3 7DR
Tel: 01865 759800
Email: info@ace-centre.org.uk
www.ace-centre.org.uk
A specialist centre focusing on the needs of those with communication deficits in both speaking and/or writing. Assessment (fee payable) can be arranged.

BECTA (British Educational Communications and Technology Agency)
Milburn Hill Road
Science Park
Coventry CV4 7JJ
Tel: 024 7641 6994
www.becta.org.uk
BECTA has a special needs team which primarily provides a service to teachers and other educational professionals.

General suppliers

AVP
School Hill Centre
Chepstow
Monmouthshire, NP16 5PH
Tel: 01291 625439
Fax: 01291 629671
Email: sales@avp.co.uk
www.avp.co.uk

The Dyscovery Centre
4a Church Road
Whitchurch
Cardiff
CF14 2DZ
Tel: 029 2062 8222
Fax: 029 2062 8333
Email: info@dyscovery.co.uk
www.dyscovery.co.uk

IANSYST
Fen House
Fen Road
Cambridge CB4 1UN
Tel: 01223 420101
Fax: 01223 426644

REM
Great Western House
Langport
Somerset TA10 9YU
Tel: 01458 254700
Fax: 01458 254701
Email: sales@r-e-m.co.uk
www.r-e-m.co.uk

The adult at work

Useful organizations

CSV (Community Service Volunteers)
Tel: 020 7278 6601
Free phone hotline for volunteers: 0800 374 991
www.csv.org.co.uk
Finds volunteering opportunities aged 16+ with free food and accommodation, plus a small weekly allowance.

www.disability.gov.uk
Provides information about the role of government in support of the interests of disabled people in the UK and Europe and provides links to other organizations representing disabled people.

Disability Rights Commission
Tel: 08457 622 633
www.drc-gb.org
The Disability Rights Commission website is a major source of information and guidance about the rights of disabled people and the duties of employers and service providers under disability legislation.

Employers' Forum on Disability
Tel: 020 7403 3020
Promotes employment for disabled people and produces various briefing papers. Briefing paper No. 6 is on Dyslexia in the Workplace. National employers' membership organization focused on training and employment of people with disabilities.
www.employers-forum.co.uk

Employment Opportunities for People with Disabilities
(Head Office)
53 New Broad Street
London EC2M 1SL
Tel: 020 7448 5420
Fax: 020 7374 4913
Email: info@eopps.org
www.opportunities.org.uk
A national charity with regional centres working with employers to help
people with disabilities to find work.

The Ergonomic Society
Website holding useful information on ergonomics in the workplace and
list of registered consultancies who are able to provide bespoke ergonomic advice on workstation design.
www.ergonomics.org.uk

Home-workers.com
www.homeworkers.com

Job Centre Plus Disability Service Team at your local Job Centre Plus
Disability Employment Advisor (DEA)
www.employmentservice.org.uk
Also www.jobcentreplus.co.uk

Mencap (Pathway to Employment Service)
Tel: 020 7454 0454
www.mencap.org.uk

The Prince's Trust
18 Park Square East
London NW1 4LH
Tel: 0800 842 842
www.princes-trust.org.uk

RADAR
Tel: 020 7250 3222
Gives advice on the Disability Discrimination Act.

Rathbone
Tel: 0161 236 5358
A training provider for young people and unemployed adults who may
have special training or educational needs. Rathbone works in partner-
ship with LEAs, businesses, charitable trusts and foundations.

Remploy
Stonecourt
Siskin Drive
Coventry CV3 4FJ
Tel: 024 7651 5800
Helpline: 0845 845 2244
Fax: 024 7651 5860
www.remploy.co.uk

Shaw Trust
Shaw House
Epsom Square
White Horse Business park
Trowbridge
Wiltshire BA14 0XJ
Tel: 01225 716350
Fax: 01225 716334
Email: stir@shaw-trust.org.uk
www.shaw-trust.org.uk
Shaw Trust is a national charity that provides training and work opportunities for people disadvantaged in the labour market through disability, ill health or other social circumstances.

Skill
Chapter House
18–20 Crucifix Lane
London SE1 3JW
www.skill.org.uk

Workable
Tel: 020 7608 3161
Offers employers specialist advice and information on disability.

The adult at play

Useful organizations

AA (Automobile Association)
Tel: 0870 5500600
Helpline: 0800 262050, Disability Helpline: 0800 262050
www.theaa.co.uk

Alexander Technique
The Society of Teachers of Alexander Technique
129 Camden Mews
London NW1 9AH
Tel: 020 7284 3338
Fax: 020 7482 5435
Email: office@stat.org.uk
Teachers of Alexander technique 0845 230 7828
www.stat.org.uk

Archery Society
National Agricultural Centre
Stoneleigh
Kenilworth
Warwickshire CV8 2LG
Tel: 024 7669 6631
Fax: 024 7641 9662
www.gnas.org

Aromatherapy
International Federation of Aromatherapists
182 Chiswick High Road
London W4 1PP
Tel: 020 8742 2605
Email: office@ifaroma.org

Aromatherapy websites:
http://www.fragrant.demon.co.uk/aroma1.html
http://www.fragrant.demon.co.uk/
http://www.kevala.co.uk/aromatherapy/index.cfm

Back2normal
Tel: 020 7357 6877
www.back2normal.co.uk

Big Print Ltd
PO Box 173
Peterborough PE2 6WS
Tel: 0800 124007
Email: bigprint@rnib.org.uk
www.big-print.co.uk

British Canoe Union
John Dudderidge House
Adbolton Lane
West Bridgford
Notts NG2 5AS
Tel: 0115 982 1100
Fax: 0115 982 1797
Email: info@bcu.org.uk

British Disabled Flying Association
Building 174
Biggin Hill Airport
Main Road
Westerham
Kent TN16 3BN
Tel: 07967 269345
Email: info@bdfa.net
www.bdfa.net

British Society for Music Therapy
61 Church Hill Road
East Barnet
Herts EN4 8SY
Tel: 020 8441 6226
Fax: 020 8441 4118
www.bsmt.org

The British Wheel of Yoga
1 Hamilton Place
Boston Road
Sleaford
Lincs NG 34 7ES
Tel: 01529 306 851

Circles Network
Pamwell House
160 Pennywell Road
Upper Easton
Bristol BS5 0TX
Tel: 0117 9393917
www.circlesnetwork.org.uk
This organization aims to support people who are isolated through disability to become included in community life.

The Department of Transport's Mobility Advice and Information Service (MAVIS)
Tel: 01344 661 000
www.mobility-unit.dtlr.gov.uk
Information about concessions on the theory test is available from:
Drive Safe
Driving Standards Agency Special Needs Team
Tel: 0870 0101 3721

Disabled Drivers' Association
Ashwellthorpe
Norwich NR16 1EX
Tel: 01508 489449
Fax: 01508 488173
Email: hq@dda.org.uk
Information on driving assessment.

Drivers Medical Group (DMG)
DVLA
Swansea SA99 1TU
Tel: 0870 600 0301
Fax: 01792 761100
Email: drivers.dvla@gtnet.gov.uk
www.dvla.gov.uk/drivers/dmed1.htm
Drivers who require information about the DVLA rules for SpLD candidates wishing to apply for a provisional licence should apply to this unit.

National Federation of Anglers
Halliday House
Egginton Junction
Derbyshire DE65 6GU
Tel: 01283 734 735
Fax: 01283 734 799
www.fire.org.uk/nfa

The National Key Scheme
Details from:
RADAR
Tel: 020 7250 3222
www.radar.org.uk
Provides access to over 5000 public toilets that might be subject to van-
dalism unless kept locked.

The National Trust
42 Queen Anne's Gate
London SW1H 9AS
Tel: 020 7222 9251
Fax: 020 7222 5097
www.nationaltrust.org.uk

National Watersports Centre
Holme Pierrepont off Regatta Way
Trent Bridge
Nottingham NG12 2LU
Tel: 0115 982 1212
www.nationalwatersports.co.uk

Outward Bound Trust
Ullswater
Watermillock
Penrith
Cumbria CA11 OJL
Tel: 01990 134 227
Fax: 01768 486983

Perfect Parking Every Time
Device aimed to help people to park when the car is near to an object.
Tel: 0871 2695

Pilates
www.bodycontrol.co.uk

The Pilates Foundation UK Ltd
PO Box 36052
London SW16 1XQ
Tel: 07071 781 859
Fax: 020 8696 0088
Email: admin@pilatesfoundation.com

Ramblers Association
1–5 Wandsworth Road
London SW8 2XX
Tel: 020 7339 8500
Fax: 020 7339 8501
Email: ramblers@london.ramblers.org.uk
www.ramblers.org.uk

Relaxation and Massage
http://www.relaxation.clara.net/
http://www.massagetherapy.co.uk
www.backpain.org

Riding for the Disabled Association
Lavinia Norfolk House
Avenue R
National Agricultural Centre
Stoneleigh Park CV8 2LY
Tel: 024 7669 6510
Fax: 024 7669 6532

Skiing
Up Hill Ski Club
www.uphillskiclub.co.uk

Tai Chi
To find your nearest Tai Chi group/course look on the web page
http://www.taichifinder.co.uk/

Talking Newspapers Association of the UK
National Recording Centre
10 Browning Road
Heathfield
East Sussex TN21 8DB
Tel: 01435 866102
Fax: 01435 865422
www.tnuk.org.uk

Thrive (Gardening)
The Geoffrey Udall Building
Trunkwell Park
Beech Hill
Reading
Berks RG7 2AT
Tel: 0115 988 5688
Fax: 0118 988 5677
Email: hort-therapy@compuserve.com
www.ourworld.compuserve.com/homepages/hort-therapy
www.carryongardening.org.uk

Tripscope
www.tripscope.org.uk
The Vassal Centre
Gill Avenue
Bristol BS16 2QQ
Tel: 08457 585641
Information service on travel and transport for people with mobility problems.

Write Away (Adults)
1 Thorpe Close
London W10 5XL
Tel: 020 8964 4225
Email: info@writeaway.demon.co.uk
This is a penfriend club.

The adult at home

Useful organizations

Disability Living Allowance Unit
Warbreck House
Warbreck Hill
Blackpool FY2 OYF
Tel: Helpline 0345 123 456

Family Therapy
24-32 Stephensons Way
London NW1 2HX
Tel: 020 7391 9150
Fax: 020 7391 9169

Relate
Herbert Grey College
Little Church Street
Rugby CV21 3AP
Tel: 0845 456 1310
Fax: 01788 535007
www.relate.org.uk
For Relate direct telephone counselling service – 0845 130 4016

Small aids and equipment

DLF (Disability Living Foundation)
380–384 Harrow Road
London W9 2HU
Helpline: 0870 6039176
www.dlf.org.uk
Impartial advice about equipment for overcoming problems in daily living experienced by people with disabilities.

Home Craft Ability One Ltd
Shelly Close
Lowmoor Road Industrial Estate
Kirkby-in-Ashfield
Nottinghamshire NG17 7ET
Tel: 01623 720005

Nottingham Rehab Supplies
Norvara House
Excelsior Road
Ashby de la Zouch
Leicestershire LE65 1NG
Tel: 0845 120 4522
Email: info@nrs-uk.co.uk
www.nrs-uk.co.uk

Posturite (UK) Ltd
10 Diplocks Way
Hailsham
East Sussex BN27 3JF
Email: support@posturite.co.uk
www.posturite.co.uk

Promedics Ltd (NorthCoast Medical)
Moorgate Street
Blackburn BB2 4PB
Tel: 01254 619000
Email: enquiries@promedics.co.uk
www.promedics.co.uk

The National Disability Helpline
Tel: 0845 1309177 9 (Mon–Fri, 10.00–16.00)
Provides advice and information on equipment and gadgets and can put
callers in touch with other organizations.

Helpful reading

Benefits Information Guide
HMSO Publications Centre
PO Box 276
London SW8 5DT
Tel: 020 7873 0011 (or from Stationery Offices)

Further reading

DCD/dyspraxia

Dyspraxia: The Hidden Handicap
Dr Amanda Kirby
Souvenir Press, 1999

Guide to Dyspraxia and Developmental Co-ordination Disorders
Amanda Kirby and Sharon Drew
David Fulton Publishers, 2003

Living with Dyspraxia: A guide for adults with developmental
Dyspraxia
Compiled by Mary Colley and The Dyspraxia Foundation Adult Support
Group
Dyspraxia Foundation Adult Support Group, 2000

Stephen Harris in Trouble
Tim Nichol
Jessica Kingsley Publishers, 2003

Dyslexia

Adult Dyslexia: A Guide for the Workplace
Gary Fitzgibbon and Brian O'Connor
Wiley, 2002

Dyslexia in Adults: Education and Employment
G Reid and J Kirk
John Wiley & Sons Ltd, 2001

Dyslexia in the Workplace
D Barlett and S Moody
Whurr Publishers, 2000

Dyslexia: Signposts to Success
J. Matty (ed.)
British Dyslexia Association, 1995

Asperger's

Asperger Syndrome and Adolescence: Practical Solutions for School
Success
Brenda Smith Myles and Diane Adreon
Autism Asperger Publishing Company, 2001

Asperger Syndrome Employment Workbook: An Employment Workbook
for Adults with Asperger Syndrome
Roger N Meyer
Jessica Kingsley Publishers, 2001

Aspergers in Love: Couple Relationships and Family Affairs
Maxine C Aston
Jessica Kingsley Publishers, 2003

Living and Loving with Asperger's Syndrome
Patrick, Estelle and Jared McCabe
Jessica Kingsley Publishers, 2003

ADHD

ADHD: Attention-Deficit Hyperactivity Disorder in Children, Adolescents
and Adults
Paul H Wender
Oxford University Press, 2001

Adult ADD, the Complete Handbook: Everything You Need to Know
About How to Cope and Live Well with ADD/ADHD
David B Sudderth et al.
Prima Publishing, 1997

Clinical Interventions for Adult ADHD: A Comprehensive Approach
Sam Goldstein and Anne Teeter Ellison
Academic Press, 2002

Family Therapy for ADHD: Treating Children, Adolescents and Adults
Craig A Everett and Sandra Volgy Everett
Guilford Press, 2001

Hyperactive Children Grown Up: ADHD in Children, Adolescents and
Adults
Gabrielle Weiss and Lily Trokenberg Hechtman
Guilford Press, 1993

Treatment and Science of Attention Deficit Disorder (ADD/ADHD) in
Adults, Teenagers and Children
M A Gross
Nova Science Publishers, 1997

General

People Skills for Young Adults
Marianna Csoti
Jessica Kingsley Publishers, 1999

You Don't Outgrow It: Living with Learning Disabilities
Marnell L Hayes, EdD
Ann Abor Publishers Ltd, 1993

Useful contacts

ADDISS (Attention Deficit Disorder Information and Support Service)
10 Station Road
Mill Hill
London NW7 2JU
Tel: 020 8906 9068
Fax: 020 8959 0727
Email: info@addiss.co.uk
www.addiss.co.uk

Adult Dyslexia Organization
336 Brixton Road
London SW9 7AA
Helpline tel: 020 7924 9559
Email: dyslexia.hq@dial.pipex.com
www.futurenet.co.uk/charity/ado/index.html

After 16, What next?
Helpline: 0845 130 4542 (Mon–Fri, 9.00–17.00)
www.after16.org.uk
www.familyfundtrust.org.uk
Gives information and advice for young disabled people.

British Association of Occupational Therapists
(College of Occupational Therapists)
106–114 Borough High Street
Southwark
London SE11LB
Tel: 020 7357 6480
www.cot.co.uk

Chartered Society of Physiotherapy
14 Bedford Row
Chancery Lane
London WC1R 4ED
Tel: 020 7306 6666
Email csp@csphysio.org.uk
www.csp.org.uk

Contact-a-Family
Tel: 0808 808 3555 (Mon–Fri, 10.00–16.00)
www.cafamily.org.uk

DANDA (Developmental Adult Neuro-Diversity Association)
46 Westbere Road
London NW2 3RU
Tel: 020 7435 7891

Dyscovery Centre
Tel: 029 2062 8222
Fax: 029 2062 8333
Email: dyscoverycentre@btclick.com
www.dyscovery.co.uk
Offers advice and information on specific learning difficulties and training
courses, seminars and lectures to managers and employers.

The Dyslexia Institute
Head Office and National Training Resource Centre
Park House
Wick Road
Egham
Surrey TW20 0HH
Tel: 01784 222 3000
Fax: 01784 222 333
Email: info@dyslexia-inst.org.uk
www.dyslexia-inst.org.uk

Dyspraxia Foundation
8 West Alley
Hitchin
Herts SG5 1EG
Tel: 01462 454986
Fax: 01462 455052
www.embrook.demon.co.uk/dyspraxia

MIND
15–19 Broadway
London E15 4BQ
Info line: 08457 660163 (Mon–Fri, 09.15–15.15)
www.mind.org.uk

The National Autistic Society
393 City Road
London EC1V 1NG
Helpline: 0845 070 4004
Information centre: info@nas.org.uk
www.nas.org.uk

Royal College of Speech and Language Therapists
2 Whiteheart Yard
London SE1 1NX
Tel: 020 7378 1200
Fax: 020 7403 7254
Email postmaster@rcslt.org
www.rcslt.org.uk

Young Minds
102–108 Clerkenwell Road
London EC1M 5SA
Tel: 020 7336 8445
Fax: 020 7336 8446
www.youngminds.org.uk

Glossary of terms

ADD:	Attention deficit disorder
ADHD:	Attention deficit hyperactivity disorder
ADL:	Activities of daily living
Apraxia:	The lack of praxis or motor planning. Interference with planning and executing an unfamiliar task
Articulation:	The production of vowels and consonants by the active and passive articulators in the mouth. The active articulators are the moving parts of the mouth (lips/tongue/soft palate) that can produce sounds whilst the passive articulators are the non-moving parts of the mouth (hard palate/teeth) against which, in the production of many sounds, the active articulators come into contact
AS:	Asperger's syndrome
ASD:	Autistic spectrum disorder
Asperger's syndrome:	A specific learning difficulty named after Hans Asperger, which results in social and communication difficulties. There is an overlap with other specific learning difficulties
Asymmetry:	One side of the body is different from the other, i.e. one side shorter or more flexed than the other
Ataxia:	Literally, disorder: applied to any defective control of muscles and consequent irregularity of movements
ATNR:	Asymmetrical Tonic Neck Reflex. A posture adopted with the head and arms in response to stretch applied to the neck muscles, e.g. when the head is turned to the left, the arm and leg on that side extend, while the limbs on the opposite side flex. It should be integrated into the movement system by 4 months of age
Atopy:	Form of allergy such as asthma, hay fever or eczema

Attention: Attention requires arousal, orientation and focus

Auditory: Pertaining to the hearing

Auditory discrimination: The ability to hear the difference between sounds that are similar to each other in terms of place and manner of production (e.g. 'f' vs 'v' – 'pat' vs 'bat')

Auditory memory: The ability to retain and recall verbal information

Auditory perceptual problems: Trouble taking information through the sense of hearing and/or processing that information

Auditory sequential memory: The ability to hear a sequence of sounds or words or sentences and be able to hold them in the memory for sufficient time to be able to gain information from them, process that information and respond to it

Autism: A learning difficulty affecting the individual's ability to communicate socially. Typically individuals display the following characteristics: prefer sameness and routine, behave in a bizarre way, handle or spin objects, do not make eye contact, do not join in with others, copy words, talk about one topic only

Balance: Ability to stay in and regain a position such as standing and sitting

Beyton score: Used as a measure of increased ligamentous laxity, e.g. as seen in Ehlers Danlos syndrome

Bilateral: Refers to the ability to co-ordinate both sides of the body.

Bilateral integration: This is the ability to move both sides of the body in opposing patterns of movement such as jumping sideways

Body percept: A person's perception of his own body; it consists of sensory pictures or 'maps' of the body stored in the brain. It may also be called the body scheme or body image

Central programming: Neural functions that are innate within the central nervous system; they do not have to be learned. Crawling on hands and knees and walking are good examples of centrally programmed actions

Cerebellar: (Cerebellum) outgrowth from the hindbrain overlying the medulla oblongata. Concerned with co-ordination of movement

Cluttering: Rapid and muddled speech

Coaching: Coaching explains and demonstrates to the individual how they can be helped, reflects on the learning and then helps to review progress and creates future plans to give a desired outcome

Co-contraction: The simultaneous contraction of all the muscles around a joint to stabilize it

Cognition:	The ability to understand/comprehend and attach relevance
Communication:	The act of conveying one's meaning to others. Communication occurs when one person's behaviour is interpreted or inferred as meaningful and understood by their partner in the interaction. Communication may be intentional or unintentional. All communication normally involves the interaction of both verbal and non-verbal components
Co-morbidity:	A situation where an individual may be suffering from two or more conditions, e.g. an individual with Asperger's syndrome may also have developmental co-ordination disorder
Co-ordination:	Muscles working together to achieve smooth, efficient movements
Cross laterality:	This is where an individual, for example, may be right-eyed, left-handed and right-footed. This is seen more often in individuals with developmental co-ordination disorder
DAMP:	Deficit of attention and motor perception
DCD:	Developmental co-ordination disorder
DEA:	Disability employment advisor – based at the job centre
Development:	Process of growth of all body parts and functions, physical, emotional and intellectual
Directional awareness:	This is the ability to move in different directions such as forwards, backwards and sideways
Distractible:	Not able to concentrate
DLA:	Disability living allowance
Dysdiadochokinesis:	Inability to carry out rapid alternating movement, such as rotating the hands
Dysarthria:	Difficulty in the articulation of speech sounds, attributable to muscular or neuromuscular defects. Dysarthria comprises a group of speech disorders resulting from disturbances in muscular control. Because there has been damage to the central or peripheral nervous system, some degree of weakness, slowness, lack of co-ordination, or altered muscle tone characterizes the activity of the speech mechanism
Dyscalculia:	A problem with mathematical concepts
Dysgraphia:	A difficulty with handwriting
Dyslexia:	Difficulty in reading or learning to read
Dysmorphic facies:	Unusual facial features
Dysphagia:	Swallowing disorders characterized by difficulty in oral preparation for the swallow or in moving a bolus from the mouth to the stomach. Subsumed in this definition are problems in positioning food in the mouth, including suckling, sucking and mastication

Dysphasia:	A disturbance of language that can affect both receptive and expressive skills, sometimes one more than the other. It can affect spoken/written/gestured language
Dyspraxia:	Poor praxis or motor planning, a less severe but more common dysfunction than apraxia
EEG:	Electro-encephalogram – this measures brain waves. Used when considering if someone has epilepsy
EFA:	Essential fatty acids
Efalex:	A fatty acid supplement prescribed to individuals with ADHD and dyspraxia
Ehlers Danlos syndrome:	A connective tissue disorder
Equilibrium:	Refers to body movements or shift in weight in order to regain/maintain balance
Expressive language:	Communication by means of the spoken word. The ability to produce spoken language that is grammatically/syntactically sound and coherent in both content and sequence
Extension:	The action of straightening, e.g. back, neck, arms or legs
Eye/hand co-ordination:	This is the ability of the eyes and hands to work together, e.g. it is needed for writing
Ey-Q:	A fatty acid supplement prescribed for individuals with ADHD and DCD/dyspraxia
Finger agnosia:	The ability to recognize which finger is being touched when vision is excluded
Flexion:	The act of bending or pulling in a part of the body
Foundation skills:	Skills required for general development, i.e. vision, balance, bilateral integration, co-ordination and motor planning. These skills are necessary at an automatic level in order to learn more complex skills
Frontal lobe:	An area of the brain that deals with integrating most of the functions of the brain, e.g. conceptualizing and planning. It also has a role in the conscious process of emotion
GDD:	Global developmental delay – this is where the individual has difficulties across all areas of learning
Grammar:	Refers to the way in which words are and can be combined to make sentences
Grapheme:	Letters of the alphabet
HFA:	Higher functioning autism
Higher level language:	The ability to process, integrate, interpret and organize verbal/written language
HUFA:	Highly unsaturated fatty acids
Hypernasal:	Excessive escape of air through the nose, producing a voice such as that often heard in people with cleft palate

Hyperpigmented macules:	Highly pigmented spots on the skin
Hyponasal:	Reduced passage of air through the nose producing a voice sounding as if the person is 'blocked up' with a bad cold
Information carrying words:	Refers to those words that carry key information within an utterance
Interdisciplinary working:	This is where team members working from different disciplines work directly with each other not just alongside
Language:	A code system used for conveying messages and sharing information among those who know the code. It may be transmitted by speech, writing or gesture. Use of language depends on a receptive channel (comprehension) and an expressive channel. Language is typically described in terms of: (i) structure: grammar (syntax), morphology (the form of words) (ii) pronunciation: phonetics, phonology (the use of sound contrasts to signal meaning) (iii) meaning: vocabulary (meanings of words), semantics, discourse (language in context; functions of language)
Lateral:	The aspect of a limb or body part furthest away from the body's midline
Laterality:	The tendency for certain processes to be handled more efficiently on one side of the brain than on the other. In most people the right hemisphere becomes more efficient in processing spatial and musical patterns, while the left specializes in verbal and logical processes
Laxity:	Lack of ligamentous support at joints allowing a wider than average range of movement
Left cerebral hemisphere:	A part of the brain that deals with detail and logic
Limbic system:	A part of the brain that controls emotion
Lumbar:	The natural curve of the lower spine
MBD:	Minimal brain disorder
Medial:	The aspect of a limb or body part closest to the body's midline
Midline:	This develops out of laterality. An individual needs to have a well defined midline in order to develop a sense of space around him and to be able to orientate himself to his surroundings
Mind mapping:	A note-taking/organizational method that is useful for visual learners
MLD:	Moderate learning difficulties
Moro reflex:	A reflex usually seen in newborn babies, but which usually disappears after first few months
Motor planning:	The ability of the brain to conceive, organize and carry out a sequence of unfamiliar actions – also known as praxis

MRI:	Magnetic resonance imaging – a type of brain scan
Multi-sensory learning:	The learner is taught through different sensory modalities, e.g. visual, auditory, kinaesthetic routes
Muscular dystrophy:	An inherited condition which affect the muscles
NDD:	Neurodevelopment delay
Neurons:	Nerve cells in the brain that carry electrical signals
NLD:	Non-verbal learning disorder
Non-verbal:	Refers to all other ways in which individuals use the context to understand what someone is saying
Nystagmus:	Irregular eye movements of the eyes
Occipital lobe:	A part of the brain that deals mainly with processing vision
OCD:	Obsessional compulsive disorder – individuals have an obsession with certain areas of their life, typically this tends to be counting, washing and checking
OP:	Occupational psychologist
Oppositional defiant disorder:	Individuals are oppositional to demands from others and show little signs of remorse when told off
Oral peripheral examination:	The passive and active oral structures are investigated to ascertain the existence of any abnormality. Their function is then determined to ascertain whether any breakdown in the accuracy/speed/sequencing/co-ordination of movement could be contributing to decreased speech intelligibility and/or exacerbating feeding patterns
PDD:	Pervasive developmental disorder
PDP:	Personal development plan
Perception:	The meaning the brain gives to sensory input
Perceptual constancy:	The ability to perceive an object as possessing certain properties such as shape, position and size in spite of the different way it may be presented
Perceptuo-motor co-ordination:	Term used to mean individuals with DCD/dyspraxia
Pes planovalgus:	A correctable foot deformity appearing as a flattening of the arches due to lack of ligamentous support and muscle strength
PET:	Positron emission tomography – a type of brain scan that produces very clear pictures
Petit mal:	A type of epilepsy. Individuals have 'absences' and lose concentration for short periods of time
Phonation:	The production of voice by the vibration of the vocal folds (cords) using exhaled air
Phoneme:	Speech sound
Phonological awareness:	The ability to identify numbers and syllables and repeat multi-syllabic words, to detect/generate rhymes, to blend and segment words into their component syllables and sounds. These skills are

important – prerequisite skills for developing reading, writing and spelling

Phonology: Refers to the rules that allow individuals to perceive and produce the differences between sounds in a highly regular manner. These rules are usually acquired within the first three or four years of age

PND: Postnatal depression

Pragmatics: Refers to the individual's ability to use language in context; when we talk about pragmatics we are always interested in the speaker and in what is said and the way it is perceived

Pronation: Downward turning of the palm of the hand.

Prone: Horizontal body position with the face and stomach downward

Proprioception: From the Latin word 'one's own'. The sensations from the muscles and joints. Proprioceptive input tells the brain when and how the joints are bending, extending or being pulled or compressed. This information enables the brain to know where each part of the body is and how it is moving

Protective extension: The reflex that extends the arms to provide protection when the body is falling

PUFA: Polyunsaturated fatty acids

Putamen: A part of the brain that looks after automatic movements, e.g. those that have been learned by repetition, and keeps them working smoothly

RA: Reading age

Raw score: Is a term used when counting the number of correct responses on a standardized test. It is usually contrasted with the standard score

Receptive language: The ability to understand language

Reflexes: Always exactly the same response to a certain stimulus e.g. turning the head to the left causes extension of the limbs on that side, and flexion of limbs on the other side

Refractive error: The lens power required producing a perfectly focused image on the retina

Right cerebral hemisphere: A part of the brain that controls emotion and sees the bigger picture. More active in females

Ritalin: A drug used in the treatment of attention deficit hyperactivity disorder

SA: Spelling age

Semantics: Refers to meaning conveyed by vocabulary and the grammatical structures that an individual uses

Sensory input: The stream of electrical impulses flowing from the sense receptors in the body to the spinal cord in the brain

Sequencing:	The ability to master individual steps in an activity and pass from one component part to the next in the correct order
Skill:	The efficiency in carrying out a task
Somasthetic:	Pertaining to the body
Spatial orientation:	Knowledge of space and the distance between the self and objects in the environment
Speech:	Spoken language – makes use of phonation and articulation
SpLD:	Specific learning difficulty
Standard score:	Is the single most important score derived from a standardized test; this allows us to express the individual's performance in terms of where it comes relative to a group of individuals on whom the test was originally developed
Stereognosis:	The ability to perceive and understand the shape and size and texture of objects by the sense of touch alone
STNR:	Symmetrical tonic neck reflex. Postures adopted by the arms and legs in response to stretch applied to the neck muscles, e.g. when the neck is extended the arms extend while the legs flex. When the head is flexed, the arms collapse into flexion and the legs extend. It should be integrated into movement by 4 months of age
Supination:	Turning the palm of the hand upward
Supine:	Horizontal body position with face and stomach upward
Symmetrical integration:	This is the ability to move both sides of the body simultaneously in identical patterns of movement. An individual should be able to jump forwards with both feet together 10 out of 10 times
Tactile defensiveness:	A sensory integrative dysfunction in which tactile sensations cause excessive emotional reactions, hyperactivity or other behavioural problems
Tic:	Abnormal facial movement that is not under the control of the individual
Tone:	The normal state of readiness of healthy muscle fibres at rest
Tourette's syndrome:	Named after Gilles de la Tourette. Uncontrollable outbursts, either physical or verbal, e.g. facial tics. The putamen (an area of the brain) is thought to be overactive and triggers the acting out of learned movements or skills at inappropriate moments
Transition:	Creating an environment where an individual can move successfully from one area to another e.g. school to further education/employment
Uni-modal learner:	The individual tends to use one sensory strategy at a time

Verbal:	Refers to the person's ability to comprehend the spoken word
Vestibular system:	The sensory input that responds to the position of the head in relation to gravity and decelerated or accelerated movement
Visual:	Pertaining to sight
Visual closure:	The ability to recognize an object when presented as an incomplete form
Visual discrimination:	The ability to discriminate similarities and differences in characteristics, arrangements, sequences, organization of visual stimuli
Visual figure ground:	The ability to differentiate stimulus from its background or the ability to attend to one stimulus without being distracted by irrelevant visual stimuli
Visual memory:	The ability to recall characteristics of stimuli through vision only.
Visual motor integration:	The integration of visual motor information that enables the eye-hand co-ordination that is required to carry out activities
Visual perception:	Judging of depth, visual closure, visual discrimination and visual figure ground i.e. processing information, seeing the difference between two objects, seeing how far and near objects might be
Visual spatial relationships:	The ability to sense the relationship of objects from each other and from oneself. Depth, length, position, direction and movement are all aspects of this sense
Winging:	Where the shoulder blades stand proud of the chest wall through lack of muscular support
WISC:	Weschler Intelligence Test – used by educational psychologists as one of the measures of intelligence
Word finding difficulties:	Individuals have difficulty thinking of the word they want to say quickly and accurately, even though they do know the word. These difficulties interrupt attempts at conversation and are frustrating for the speaker as well as the listener

Tests

Physical/motor skills

Test	Supplier
Crawfords Small Parts Dexterity Test	The Psychological Corporation Harcourt Education Halley Court Jordans Hill Oxford OX2 8EJ Tel: 44 (0) 1865 888188 www.tpc-international.com
Fine Dexterity Test	Educational and Industrial Test Services Ltd 83 High Street Hemel Hempstead Herts HP13AH UK
Grooved Peg Board Test	www.rehaboutlet.com
Two Arm Co-ordination Test	www.rehaboutlet.com
The Quick Neurological Screening Test II (1998) Revision	Ann Arbor Publishers Ltd PO Box 1 Belford Northumberland NE70 7JX Tel: 44 (0) 1668214460 www.annarbor.co.uk
Aston Postural Assessment Judith Aston 1998	Psychological Corporation

Independent living skills

Test	Supplier
The Assessment of Motor and Process Skills (AMPS) AG Fisher, 1999 (Accredited Use Required)	AMPS UK Tel: 01225 864847 Email: info@amps-uk.com
Canadian Occupational Performance Measure (3rd edn) Mary Law et al., 1998	Canadian Association of Occupational Therapists (800) 434-2268 ext 242 Email: publications@caot.ca www.caot.ca

Visual

Test	Supplier
Beery Buktenica Developmental Test of Visual Motor Integration Keith Beery and Norman Buktenica	Ann Arbor Publishers Ltd
Test of Visual Motor Skills (12–40 years) TVMS (UL) Morrison F Gardner	Ann Arbor Publishers Ltd
Motor-Free Visual Perception Test (MVPT-3) Ronald P Calarusso and Donald D Hammill	Ann Arbor Publishers Ltd
Test of Visual Perceptual Skills (Non Motor) Upper Level – Revised TVPS-UL-R Morrison F Gardner	Ann Arbor Publishers Ltd
Developmental Test of Visual Perception – Adolescent and Adult (DTVP-A) Cecil R Reynolds, Nils A Pearson and Judith K Voress, 2002	The Psychological Corporation

Language

Test	Supplier
Test of Auditory Perceptual Skills – Upper Level (12–18 years) Morrison F Gardner	Ann Arbor Publishers Ltd

Test of Adolescent and Adult
Language – 3rd Edition
Donald D Hammill, Virginia L Brown,
Stephen C Larsen and J Lee
Wiederholt, 1994

The Psychological Corporation

Test of Adolescent/Adult Word
Finding (TAWF)
Diane J German, 1989

The Psychological Corporation

Assessment of Language Related
Functional Activities (ALFA)
Kathleen Baines, Ann W Martin
and Heidi McMartin Heeringa, 1999

The Psychological Corporation

SCAN-A: A Test for Auditory
Processing Disorders in Adults
Robert W Keith, 1994

The Psychological Corporation

Wide Range Achievement Test
3 (WRAT3)
Gary S Wilkinson, 1993

The Psychological Corporation

Cognitive/memory

Test

Supplier

Wechsler Adult Intelligence Scale –
3rd Edition (WAIS-3)
David Wechsler, 1999

The Psychological Corporation

Wide Range Achievement Test
3(WRAT3)
Gary S Wilkinson, 1993

The Psychological Corporation

Organization/attention

Test

Supplier

Brown Attention-Deficit Disorder Scales
Thomas E Brown, 2001

The Psychological Corporation

Behavioural Assessment of the
Dysexecutive Syndrome (BADS)
Barbara A Wilson, Nick Alderman,
Paul Burgess, Hazel Emslie, Jonathan J
Evans, 1996

Thames Valley Test Company
Unit 32 The Granary
Station Hill
Thurston
Bury St Edmunds
Suffolk IP31 3QU
Tel: 44 (0) 1359 232941
www.tvtc.com

| Wisconsin Card Sorting Task (WCST-64) Susan K Kongs, Laetitia L Thompson, Grant l Iverson and Robert K Heaton, 2000 | The Psychological Corporation |

Social/emotional interpersonal

Test	**Supplier**
Adaptive Behaviour Assessment System (ABAS) Patti Harrison and Thomas Oakland, 2000	The Psychological Corporation
Becks Depression Inventory – II (BDI – II) Aaron T Beck, Robert A Steer and Gregory K Brown, 1996	The Psychological Corporation
Becks Anxiety Inventory (BAI) Aaron T Beck, Robert A Steer and Gregory K Brown, 1990	The Psychological Corporation
Inventory of Interpersonal Problems (IIP-32/IIP-64) Leonard M Horowitz, Lynn E Alden, Jerry S Wigins and Aaron L Pincus, 2000	The Psychological Corporation
The Pragmatics Profile Adolescents and Adults Hazel Dewart and Susie Summers, 1996	NFER Email: information@nfer-nelson.co.uk Customer Support: 0845 6021937 www.nfer-nelson.co.uk
Social Use of Language Programme Wendy Rinaldi	NFER
The Awareness of Social Interference Test (TASIT) Skye McDonald, Sharon Flanagan, Jennifer Rollins, 2002	Thames Valley Test Company
Harter's Self-Perception Profile Adolescents and Adults Susan Harter, 1985	University of Denver Department of Psychology 2155 SO Race Street Denver Colorado 80208

References

American Psychiatric Association (1994) DSM IV. Diagnostic and Statistical Manual of Mental Disorders 53–55. 4th Revised edn. Washington: APA.

Aram DM, Horwitz SJ (1983) Sequential and non speech praxic abilities in developmental verbal apraxia. Developmental Medicine and Child Neurology 25: 197–206.

Archer LA, Witelson SF (1988) Manual motor functions in developmental dysphasia. Journal of Clinical and Experimental Neuropsychology 10: 47.

Ayres AJ (1972a) Sensory Integration and Learning Disorders. Los Angeles: Western Psychological Press.

Ayres AJ (1972b) Types of sensory integration dysfunction amongst disabled learners. American Journal of Occupational Therapy 26: 13–18.

Ayres AJ (1979) Sensory Integration and the Child. Los Angeles: Western Psychological Press.

Ayres AJ (1980) Sensory Integration and Learning Disorders. Los Angeles: Western Psychological Corporation.

Ayres AJ (1985) Developmental Dyspraxia and Adult Onset Apraxia. Torrance, CA: Sensory Integration International.

Ayres AJ, Mailloux ZK, Wendler CL (1987) Developmental dyspraxia: is it a unitary function? Occupational Therapy Journal of Research 7: 93–110.

Bairstow PJ, Laslow JI (1981) Kinaesthetic sensitivity to passive movements in children and adults and its relationship to motor development and motor control. Developmental Medicine and Child Neurology 23: 606–16.

Barkley RA, Dupaul GJ, McMurray MB (1990) A comprehensive evaluation of attention deficit disorder with and without hyperactivity. Journal of Consulting and Clinical Psychology 58: 775–89.

Barnett AL, Kooistra L, Henderson SE (1998) 'Clumsiness' as a syndrome and symptom. Human Movement Science 17: 435–47.

Blondis TA (1999) Motor disorders and attention-deficit/hyperactivity disorder. Pediatric Clinical North America 46: 899–913.

Borstein RA (1990) Neuropsychological performance in children with Tourette's syndrome. Psychiatry Research 33: 73–81.

Borstein RA, Yang V (1991) Neuropsychological performance in medicated and un-medicated patients with Tourette's disorder. American Journal of Psychiatry 148: 468–71.

Bouffard M, Watkinson EJ, Thompson LP et al. (1996) A test of the activity deficit hypothesis with children with movement difficulties. Adapted Physical Activity Quarterly 13: 61–73.

Bruininks RH (1978) Bruininks-Oseretsky Test of Motor Proficiency: Examiners Manual. Circle Pines, MN: American Guidance Service.

Bundy A (2002) Play with children with DCD: what we know, what we suspect. 5th Biennial Conference Developmental Co-ordination Disorders, Banff, Alberta, Canada.

Cantell MH (1998) Developmental co-ordination disorder in adolescence: perceptual motor academic and social outcome of early motor delay. Research Reports on Sport & Health 112. Likes – Research Centre For Sport & Health Science: Jyvaskyla, Finland.

Cantell MH, Smyth MM, Ahonen TP (1994) Clumsiness in adolescence. educational, motor, and social outcomes of motor delay detected at 5 years. Adapted Physical Activity Quarterly 11: 115–29.

Case-Smith J (1998) Defining the early intervention process. In J Case-Smith (ed.), Pediatric Occupational Therapy and Early Intervention. Boston, MA: Butterworth-Heinemann.

Casperson CJ, Powell KE, Christenson GM (1985) Physical activity, exercise and physical fitness. Definitions and distinctions for health-related research. Public Health Reports 100(2): 126–31.

Cermak SA (1985) Developmental dyspraxia. In EA Roy (ed.), Neuropsychological Studies of Apraxia and Related Disorders (pp. 115–248). Amsterdam, Netherlands: Elsevier (North Holland).

Cermak SA (1991) Somatodyspraxia. In AG Fisher, EA Murray, AC Bundy (eds), Sensory Integration – Theory and Practice. Philadelphia: F.A. Davis Co.

Cermak SA, Larkin D (2002), Developmental Co-ordination Disorder. Canada: Delmar.

Cermak SA, Coster W, Drake C (1980) Representational and non representational gestures in boys with learning difficulties. American Journal of Occupational Therapy 34: 19–26.

Cermak SA, Ward EA, Ward LM (1986) The relationship between articulation disorders and motor co-ordination in children. American Journal of Occupational Therapy 40: 546–50.

Chu S (2002) Course Notes – Occupational Therapy For Children With Developmental Co-ordination Disorder.

Clark T (2003) Post 16 provision for those with autistic spectrum conditions: some implications of the Special Educational Need and Disability Act 2001 and the Special Needs Code of Practice for Schools. Support for Learning 18(4): 184–9.

Clarkin JF, Kendall PC (1992) Co-morbidity and treatment planning: summary and future directions. Journal of Consulting and Clinical Psychology 60: 904–8.

Clifford LD (1985) A Profile of Leisure Pursuits of Seven Awkward Children. Unpublished Master's Thesis, University of Alberta, Edmonton, Alberta Canada.

Colley M (2000) Living with Dyspraxia. Herts: The Dyspraxia Foundation.

Cooke RWI, Abernethy LJ (1999) Cranial magnetic resonance imaging and school performance in very low birth weight infants and adolescence. Archives of Disease in Childhood Fetal Neonatal Edition 81: F11–F121.

David R, Deuel R, Ferry P et al. (1981) Task force on neurology of disorders of higher cerebral function in children. Child Neurology Society. Unpublished Manuscript.

Davies M, Rinaldi M (2004) Using an evidence-based approach to enable people with mental health problems to gain and retain employment, education and voluntary work. British Journal of Occupational Therapy 76(7): 319–22.

Dawdy SC (1981) Pediatric neuropsychology: caring for the developmentally dyspraxic child. Clinical Neuropsychology 3(1): 30–7.

Denckla MB (1984) Developmental dyspraxia: the clumsy child. In MD Levine, P Satz (eds), Middle Childhood: Development and Dysfunction. Baltimore, MD: University Park Press.

Denckla MB, Roeltgen DP (1992) Disorders of motor function and control. In I Rapin, SJ Segalowitz (eds), Handbook of Neuropsychology. Amsterdam: Elsevier Science.

Denckla MB, Harris EL, Aylward EH et al. (1991) Executive functions and volume of the basal ganglia in children with Tourette's syndrome and attention deficit hyperactivity disorder. Annals of Neurology 30: 476.

Deuel PK, Doar BP (1992) Developmental manual dyspraxia: a lesson in mind and brain. Journal of Child Neurology 7: 99–103.

Dewey D (1995) What is developmental dyspraxia? Brain and Cognition 29: 254–74.

Dewey D, Wilson BN (2001) Developmental co-ordination disorder; what is it? In C Missiuna (ed.), Children with Developmental Co-ordination Disorder: Strategies for Success. New York: Hawthorn Press.

Dewey D, Roy EA., Square-Storer PA et al. (1988) Limb and oral praxic abilities in children with verbal sequencing difficulties. Developmental Medicine and Child Neurology 30: 743–51.

DfES (Department for Education and Skills) (2001) Special Educational Needs and Disability Act 2001. Nottingham: DfES Publications.

DfES (Department for Education and Skills) (2003) Bridging the Gap: A Guide to the Disabled Students Allowances (DSAs). Nottingham: DfES Publications.

Drew SA (2001) The role of the occupational therapist working with adults with DCD. Paper presentation, College of Occupational Therapist Conference, University of Swansea.

Drew SA (2002) Life skills and the adolescent with DCD. Paper presentation, Dyspraxia Professional Conference, University Of Sussex.

Eckersley J (2004) Coping with Dyspraxia. London: Sheldon Press.

Fisher AG (1998) Uniting practice and theory: an occupational framework Eleanor Clarke Slagle Lecture). American Journal of Occupational Therapy 52: 509–21.

Ford DR (1966) Diseases of the Nervous System in Infancy, Childhood and Adolescence (5th edn). Springfield, IL: Thomas.

Fox AM (1998) Clumsiness in Children. From webmaster@orcn.ahs.ca

Fox AM, Lent B (1996) Clumsy children primer on developmental co-ordination disorder. Canadian Family Physician 42: 1965–71.

Fox AM, Polatajko HJ (1994) 'The London Consensus' – From Children and Clumsiness: An International Consensus Meeting. London, Ontario, Canada, 11–14 October 1994.

Gentle AM (1992) The nature of skills acquisition: therapeutic implications for children with movement disorders. Medical Sports Science 49: 619–627.

Gerber PJ, Ginsberg R, Reiff HB (1992) Identifying alterable patterns in employment success for highly successful adults with learning disabilities. Journal of Learning Disabilities 25(8): 475–87.

Geuze RH, Borger H (1993) Children who are clumsy: five years later. Adapted Physical Activity Quarterly 10: 10–21.

Geuze RH, Kalverboer AF (1987) Inconsistency and adaptation in timing of clumsy children. Journal of Human Movement Studies 13: 421–32.

Gillberg IC, Gillberg C (1989) Children with preschool minor neurodevelopmental disorders. IV: Behaviour and school achievement at age 13. Developmental Medicine and Child Neurology 31: 3–13.

Gillberg IC, Gillberg C, Groth J (1989) Children with preschool minor neurodevelopmental disorders V: Neurodevelopmental profiles at age 13. Developmental Medicine and Child Neurology 31: 14–24.

Grove B, Giraud-Saunders A (2003) Connecting with connexions: the role of the personal adviser with young people with special educational and support needs. Support for Learning 8(1): 12–16.

Gubbay SS (1975) The Clumsy Child. New York: W.B. Saunders.

Gubbay SS (1978) The management of developmental dyspraxia. Developmental Medicine and Child Neurology 20: 643–6.

Gubbay SS (1985) Clumsiness. In PJ Vinken, GW Bruyn, Hl Klawans (eds), Handbook of Clinical Neurology (Ref Series), pp. 159–67. New York: Elsevier.

Gubbay SS (1995) The Clumsy Child: A Study of Apraxia and Agnosic Ataxia. London: Saunders.

Gubbay SS, Ellis E, Walton JN et al. (1965) Clumsy children: a study of apraxic and agnosic defects in 21 children. Brain 88: 295–312.

Hagedorn R (2001) Occupational Therapy Perspectives and Processes. London: Churchill Livingstone.

Hamilton SS (2002) Evaluation of clumsiness in young children. Journal of the American Academy of Family Physicians. www.aafp.org/afp/20021015/1435.html

Hartsough CS, Lambert NM (1985) Medical factors in hyperactive and normal children: pre-natal, developmental, and health history finding. American Journal of Orthopsychiatry 55: 190–210.

Hatton A (2004) DANDA Newsletter, Issue 2.

Hazel JS, Schumaker JB (1988) Social skills and learning disabilities: current issues and recommendations for future research. In JF Kavanaugh, TT Truss (eds), Learning Disabilities: Proceedings of the National Conference (pp. 293–344). Parkton, MD: York Press.

Hellgren L, Gillberg C, Gillberg IC et al. (1993) Children with deficits in attention, motor control and perception (DAMP), almost grown up: general health at 16 years. Developmental Medicine and Child Neurology 35: 881–92.

Hellgren L, Gillberg IC, Bagenholm A et al. (1994) Children with deficits in attention, motor control and perception (DAMP) almost grown up: psychiatric and personality disorders at age 16 years. Journal of Child Psychology and Psychiatry 35: 1255–71.

Henderson SE, Barnett AL (1998) The classification of specific motor co-ordination disorders in children: some problems to be solved. Human Movement Science 17: 449–70.

Henderson SE, Hall D (1982) Concomitants of clumsiness in young school children. Developmental Medicine and Child Neurology 24: 448–60.

Henderson SE, Sugden D (1992) Movement ABC Battery for Children Manual. Sidcup, Kent: The Psychological Corporation.

Hill EL (1998) A dyspraxic deficit in specific language impairment and developmental co-ordination disorder? evidence from hand and arm movements. Developmental Medicine and Child Neurology 40: 388–95.

HMSO (1995) The Disability Discrimination Act. London: Crown Publishing.

HMSO (1998) The Data Protection Act. London: Crown Publishing.

Honey P, Mumford A (1986) The Manual of Learning Styles. Maidenhead: Honey.

Horak FB, Shumway-Cook A, Crowe TK et al. (1988) Vestibular function and motor proficiency of children with impaired hearing or learning disability and motor impairment. Developmental Medicine and Child Neurology 30: 64–79.

Illingworth RS (1968) Delayed Motor Development. Pediatric Clinics Of North America 15: 569–80.

Jahoda M (1979) The impact of unemployment in the 1930's and the 1970's. Bulletin of the British Psychological Society 32: 309–14.

Jongmans MJ, Henderson SE, De Vries L et al. (1993) Duration of six periventricular densities in preterm infants and neurological outcome at six years of age. Archives Of Diseases in Childhood 69: 9–13.

Jongmans MJ, Henderson SE, De Vries L et al. (1998) Perceptual motor difficulties and their concomitants in six-year old children born prematurely. Human Movement Science 17: 629–53.

Kadesjo B, Gillberg C (1999) Developmental coordination disorder in Swedish 7-year-old children. Journal of American Child and Adolescent Psychiatry 38(7): 820–8.

Kalverboer AF, De Vries HJ, van Dellen T (1990) Social behaviour in clumsy children as rated by parents and teachers. In AF Kalverboer (ed.), Developmental Biopsychology. Experimental and Observational Studies in Children at Risk (pp. 257–69). Ann Arbor: University of Michigan Press.

Kaplan BJ, Wilson BN, Dewey DM et al. (1998) DCD may not be a discrete disorder. Human Movement Science 17: 471–90.

Keogh JF, Sugden D, Reynard CL et al. (1979) Identification of clumsy children: comparisons and comments. Journal of Human Movement Studies 5: 32–41.

Kirby A, Drew SA (2002) Guide to Dyspraxia and Developmental Co-ordination Disorders. London: Fulton Publishers.

Knuckey NW, Gubbay SS (1983) Clumsy children: a prognostic study. Australian Pediatric Journal 19: 9–13.

Kolb B (1999) Synaptic plasticity and the organisation of behaviour after early and late brain injury. Canadian Journal of Experimental Psychology 53: 62–75.

Larkin D, Parker HE (1999) Physical activity profiles of adolescents who experienced motor learning difficulties. In D Drouin, C Lepine, C Simard (eds), Proceedings of the 11th International Symposium for Adapted Physical Activity, pp. 175–81. Quebec, Canada.

Laslow JL, Bairstow PJ (1983) Kinaesthesis: its measurement training and relationship to motor control. Quarterly Journal of Experimental Psychology 35: 411–21.

Laszlo JL, Sainsbury KM (1993) Perceptual-motor development and prevention of clumsiness. Psychological Research 55: 167–74.

Laszlo JL, Bairstow PJ, Bartrip J et al. (1988) Clumsiness or perceptuomotor dysfunction? In AM Colley, JR Beech (eds), Cognition and Action in Skilled Behaviour. Amsterdam: Elsevier Science Publishers, pp. 293–309.

Lennox L, Cermak SA, Koomer J (1988) Praxis and gesture comprehension in 4-5 and 6 year olds. American Journal of Occupational Therapy 42: 99–104.

Levine MD (1984) Cumulative developmental debts; their impact on productivity in late middle childhood. In MD Levine, P Satz (eds), Middle Childhood: Development and Dysfunction. Baltimore, MD: University Park Press.

Levine MD (1987) Motor implementation. In MD Levine (ed.), Developmental Variation and Learning Disorders. Cambridge, MA: Educators Publishing Service, pp. 208–40.

Levine MD (1996) The Paediatric Examination of Educational Readiness at Middle Childhood (PEERAMID2) Cambridge, Mass: Educators Publishing Service, Inc.

Lewis G, Slogett A (1998) Suicide, deprivation and unemployment: record linkage study. British Medical Journal 317: 1283–86.

Losse A, Henderson SE, Elliman D et al. (1991) Clumsiness in children – do they grow out of it? A 10-year follow-up study. Developmental Medicine and Child Neurology 33: 55–68.

Lundy-Ekman L, Ivry R, Keele SW et al. (1991) Timing and force control deficits in clumsy children. Journal of Cognitive Neuroscience 3: 367–76.

McLoughlin D, Leather C, Stringer P (2002) The Adult Dyslexic: Interventions and Outcomes. London: Whurr Publishers.

Maeland AF (1992) Handwriting and perceptual-motor skills in clumsy, dysgraphic, and normal children. Perceptual and Motor Skills 75: 1207–17.

Mandich AD, Polatajko H, Missiuna C et al. (2001) Treatment of children with developmental co-ordination disorder: what is the evidence? Physical and Occupational Therapy in Pediatrics 20(2/3): 51–68.

Marlow N, Roberts BL, Cooke RWI (1993) Outcome at 8 years for children of birth weights of 1250g or less. Archives of Diseases in Childhood 68: 286–90.

Martini R, Heath N, Missiuna C (1999) A North American analysis of the relationship between learning disabilities and developmental co-ordination disorder. International Journal of Learning Disabilities 14: 46–58.

Mellard DF, Hazel SJ (1992) Social competencies as a pathway to successful life transitions. Learning Disability Quarterly 15: 251–71.

Missiuna C (2001) Children with Developmental Co-ordination Disorder: Strategies for Success. USA: The Haworth Medical Press.

Missiuna C, Polatajko HJ (1995) Developmental dyspraxia by any other name. American Journal of Occupational Therapy 49: 619–28.

Mosey AC (1993) Introduction to cognitive rehabilitation – working taxonomies. In CB Royeen (ed.), AOTA. Self Study Series: Cognitive Rehabilitation. Rockville, MD: American Occupational Therapy Association, Inc.

Mulderij KJ (1996) Research into the life world of physically disabled children. Child: Care, Health and Development 22(5): 311–22.

Murphy JB, Gliner JA (1988) Visual and Motor Sequencing in Normal and Clumsy Children. Occupational Therapy Journal of Research 8: 89–103.

National Adult Literacy and Learning Disabilities (1999) Bridges To Practice: A Research-Based Guide For Literacy Practitioners Serving Adults With Learning Disabilities, Guidebook 1, pp. 27–30.

O'Beirne C, Larkin D, Cable T (1994) Co-ordination problems and anaerobic performance in children. Adapted Physical Activity Quarterly 11: 141–9.

O'Brien V, Cermak SA, Murray E (1988) The relationship between visual-perceptual motor abilities and clumsiness in children with and without learning disabilities. American Journal of Occupational Therapy 42: 359–63.

Orton ST (1937) Reading, Writing and Speech Problems in Children. New York: Norton.

Piek JP, Skinner RA (1999) Timing and force control during a sequential tapping task in children with and without motor co-ordination problems. Journal of International Neuropsychological Society.

Polatajko HJ, Law M, Miller J et al. (1991) The effect of a sensory integration programme on academic achievement, motor performance, and self-esteem in children identified as learning disabled: results of a clinical trial. Occupational Therapy Journal of Research 11: 155–76.

Polgar S, Thomas SA (1991) Introduction to Research in the Health Sciences. Edinburgh: Churchill Livingstone.

Portwood M (2000) Understanding Developmental Dyspraxia. London: David Fulton Publishers.

Primeau L (1992) Game playing behaviour in children with developmental dyspraxia, Unpublished masters dissertation, University Of Southern California.

Regehr S, Kaplan BJ (1988) Reading disability with motor problems: can it be an inherited subtype? Pediatrics 82: 204–10.

Revie G, Larkin D (1993) Task specific intervention with children reduces movement problems. Adapted Physical Activity 10: 29–34.

Rizzolatti G, Luppino G, Matelli M (1998) The Organisation of the Cortical Motor System: New Concepts. Electroencephalography and Clinical Neurophysiology 106: 283–96.

Rose B, Larkin D, Berger, B.G. (1997) Co-ordination and gender influences on the perceived competence of children. Adapted Physical Activity Quarterly 14: 130–40.

Rowe JB, Frackowiak RSJ (1999) The impact of brain imaging technology in our understanding of motor function and dysfunction. Current Opinion in Neurobiology 9: 728–34.

Rutter M (1978) Developmental issues and prognosis. In M Rutter, E Schopler (eds), Autism: Reappraisal of Concepts and Treatment, pp. 497–505. New York: Plenum Press.

Schoemaker MM, Kalverboer AF (1994) Social and affective problems of children who are clumsy: how early do they begin? Adapted Physical Activity Quarterly 11: 130–40.

Sellers JS (1995) Clumsiness: review of causes, treatments and outlook. Pediatric Physical and Occupational Therapy 15: 39–55.

Shafer D, Schonfield I, O'Connor PA et al. (1986) Neurological soft signs and their relationship to psychiatric disorder and intelligence in childhood and adolescence. Archives of General Psychiatry 42: 343–51.

Skinner RA, Piek JP (2001). Psychosocial implications of poor motor co-ordination in children and adolescents. Human Movement Science 20: 73–94.

Smith CM (1987) Career preparation for the learning disabled. Learning Disabilities Magazine 39: 39–41.

Smyth MM, Glencross DJ (1986) Information processing deficits in clumsy children. Australian Journal of Psychology 38: 13–22.

Smyth MM, Mason UC (1997) Planning and execution of action in children with and without developmental co-ordination disorder. Journal of Child Psychology & Psychiatry 8: 1023–37.

Smyth MM, Mason UC (1998) Use of proprioception in normal and clumsy children. Developmental Medicine & Child Neurology 40: 672–81.

Soorani-Lunsing RJ, Hadders-Algra M, Olinga AA et al. (1993) Is minor neurological dysfunction at 12 years related to behaviour and cognition? Developmental Medicine and Child Neurology 35: 321–30.

Stafford I (2000) Children with movement difficulties: primary education and the development of performance indicators. British Journal of Special Education 27(2).

Stordy BJ (2000) Dark adaptation, motor skills, docosahexaenoic acid, and dyslexia. American Journal of Clinical Nutrition 71 (Suppl. S), 323S–26S.

Sugden DA, Keogh JF (1990) Problems In Movement Skill Development. Columbia, SC: University Of South Carolina.

Szatmari P, Offard DR, Boyle MH (1989) Correlates, associated impairment, and patterns of service utilisation of children with attention deficit disorder: findings from the Ontario Child Health Study. Journal of Child Psychology and Psychiatry 30: 205–17.

Taber C (1997) Taber's Cyclopedic Medical Dictionary (18th edn). Philadelphia: F.A. Davies.

Taft LT, Barowsky EL (1989) Clumsy child. Pediatric Review 10: 247–53.

Thal D, Tobias S, Morrison D (1991) Language and gesture in late talkers: a 1 year follow up. Journal of Speech & Hearing Research 34: 604–12.

Touwen BCL (1979) The examination of the child with minor neurological dysfunction. Clinics in Developmental Medicine, No 71. London: S.I.M.P with Heinemann Medical.

Touwen BCL (1990) Variability and stereotypy of spontaneous motility as predictor of neurological development of preterm infants. Developmental Medicine and Child Neurology 32: 501–8.

Turner A (1987) The principles of activities of daily living. In A Turner (ed.), The Practice of Occupational Therapy. New York: Churchill Livingstone.

van Dellen T, Geuze KH (1988) Motor response programming in clumsy children. Journal of Child Psychology and Psychiatry 29: 489–500.

Visser J, Geuze RH, Kalverboer AF (1998) The relationship between physical growth, the level of activity and the development of motor skills in adolescence: differences between children with DCD and controls. Human Movement Science 17: 573–608.

Walton JN, Ellis E, Court SDM (1962) Clumsy children: developmental apraxia and agnosia. Brain 85: 603–12.

Warr P (1984) Job loss, unemployment and psychological well-being. In VL Allen, E van der Vliert (eds), Role Transitions. New York: Plenem Press.

Wegner LM (1997) Gross motor dysfunction: its evaluation and management. In MD Levine, WB Carey, AC Crocker (eds), Developmental-Behavioural Pediatrics. 3rd edn. Philadelphia: Saunders, pp. 452–6.

Werenowska N (ed.) (2003) Dyspraxic Voices. London: DANDA, p. 16.

Wetton P (1997) Physical Education in the Early Years. London: Routledge.

White WJ (1992) The post-school adjustment of persons with learning disabilities: current status and future projections. Journal of Learning Disabilities 25(7): 448–56.

Williams HG, Woolacott MH, Ivry R (1992) Timing and motor control in clumsy children. Journal of Motor Behaviour 24: 165–72.

Willingham DB (1998) A neuropsychological theory of motor skill learning. Psychological Bulletin 105: 558–84.

Willoughby C, Polatajko HJ (1995) Motor problems in children with developmental co-ordination disorder: review of literature. American Journal of Occupational Therapy 49: 787–94.

Wilson PH, McKensie BE (1998) Information processing deficits associated with developmental co-ordination disorder: a meta-analysis of research findings. Journal of Child Psychology and Psychiatry 39: 829–40.

Wing L (1981) Asperger's syndrome: a clinical account. Psychological Medicine 11: 115–29.

Wolff PH, Melngailis I, Obregon M et al. (1995) Family patterns of developmental dyslexia. Part II: Behavioural phenotypes. American Journal of Medical Genetics (Neuropsychiatric Genetics) 60: 494–505.

World Health Organization (1992) International Classification Of Diseases – 10th edn (ICD 10). Geneva: WHO.

World Health Organization (1997) ICIDH-2: International Classification of Impairments, Activities and Participation: A manual of dimensions of disablement and functioning. Geneva: World Health Organization.

World Health Organization (2001) WHO Publishes New Guidelines to Measure Health. www.who.int/int-pr2001/en/pr2001-48.html.

Index

157